D1374331

BLACKWELL

UNDERGROUND
CLINICAL
VIGNETTES

PATHOPHYSIOLOGY III:
CVS, DERMATOLOGY, GU,
GENERAL SURGERY, 4E

BLACKWELL

UNDERGROUND CLINICAL VIGNETTES

PATHOPHYSIOLOGY III: CVS, DERMATOLOGY, GU, GENERAL SURGERY, 4E

VIKAS BHUSHAN, MD
Series Editor
University of California, San Francisco, Class of 1991
Diagnostic Radiologist

VISHAL PALL, MD MPH
Series Editor
Internist and Preventive Medicine Specialist
Government Medical College, Chandigarh – Panjab University – India, Class of 1997
Graduate School of Biomedical Sciences at UTMB Galveston, MPH, Class of 2004

TAO LE, MD
University of California, San Francisco, Class of 1996

HUI J JENNY CHEN
David Geffen School of Medicine at UCLA, Class of 2005

VANEESH SONI
University of Michigan, Ann Arbor, Class of 2006

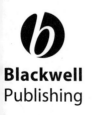

Blackwell
Publishing

Blackwell Publishing, Inc., 350 Main Street, Malden, Massachusetts 02148-5018, USA
Blackwell Publishing Ltd, 9600 Garsington Road, Oxford OX4 2DQ, UK
Blackwell Publishing Asia Pty Ltd, 550 Swanston Street, Carlton, Victoria 3053, Australia

05 06 07 08 5 4 3 2 1

ISBN-13: 978-1-4051-0416-6
ISBN-10: 1-4051-0416-3

Library of Congress Cataloging-in-Publication Data

Pathophysiology. CVS, dermatology, GU, general surgery / authors, Vikas Bhushan . . . [et al.].— 4th ed.
    p. ; cm. — (Blackwell underground clinical vignettes)
    Rev. ed. of: Pathophysiology, v. 1 / Vikas Bhushan. 3rd ed. c2002.
    ISBN-13: 978-1-4051-0416-6 (pbk. : alk. paper)
    ISBN-10: 1-4051-0416-3 (pbk. : alk. paper) 1. Cardiovascular system—Diseases—Case studies.
    [DNLM: 1. Cardiovascular Diseases—Case Reports. 2. Cardiovascular Diseases—Problems
and Exercises. WG 18.2 C2735 2005] I. Bhushan, Vikas. II. Bhushan, Vikas. Pathophysiology.
III. Series: Blackwell's underground clinical vignettes.

    RC669.9.C345 2005
    616.1—dc22

                                                                              2005003548

A catalogue record for this title is available from the British Library\

Acquisitions: Nancy Anastasi Duffy
Development/Production: Jennifer Kowalewski
Interior and Cover design: Leslie Haimes
Typesetter: Graphicraft in Quarry Bay, Hong Kong
Printed and bound by Capital City Press in Berlin, VT

For further information on Blackwell Publishing, visit our website:
www.blackwellmedstudent.com

NOTICE

The indications and dosages of all drugs in this book have been recommended in the medical literature and conform to the practices of the general community. The medications described do not necessarily have specific approval by the Food and Drug Administration for use in the diseases and dosages for which they are recommended. The package insert for each drug should be consulted for use and dosage as approved by the FDA. Because standards for usage change, it is advisable to keep abreast of revised recommendations, particularly those concerning new drugs.

The authors of this volume have taken care that the information contained herein is accurate and compatible with the standards generally accepted at the time of publication. Nevertheless, it is difficult to ensure that all the information given is entirely accurate for all circumstances. The publisher and authors do not guarantee the contents of this book and disclaim any liability, loss, or damage incurred as a consequence, directly or indirectly, of the use and application of any of the contents of this volume.

The publisher's policy is to use permanent paper from mills that operate a sustainable forestry policy, and which has been manufactured from pulp processed using acid-free and elementary chlorine-free practices. Furthermore, the publisher ensures that the text paper and cover board used have met acceptable environmental accreditation standards.

CONTENTS

CONTRIBUTORS ix

ACKNOWLEDGMENTS x

HOW TO USE THIS BOOK xii

ABBREVIATIONS xiii

CARDIOLOGY

Case 1   1
Case 2   2
Case 3   3
Case 4   4
Case 5   5
Case 6   6
Case 7   7
Case 8   8
Case 9   9
Case 10   10
Case 11   11
Case 12   12
Case 13   13
Case 14   14
Case 15   15
Case 16   16
Case 17   17
Case 18   18
Case 19   19
Case 20   20
Case 21   21
Case 22   22
Case 23   23
Case 24   24
Case 25   25
Case 26   26
Case 27   27
Case 28   28
Case 29   29

DERMATOLOGY

Case 30	30
Case 31	31
Case 32	32
Case 33	33
Case 34	34
Case 35	35
Case 36	36
Case 37	37
Case 38	38
Case 39	39
Case 40	40
Case 41	41
Case 42	42
Case 43	43
Case 44	44
Case 45	45
Case 46	46
Case 47	47
Case 48	48
Case 49	49
Case 50	50

NEPHROLOGY/UROLOGY

Case 51	51
Case 52	52
Case 53	53
Case 54	54
Case 55	55
Case 56	56
Case 57	57
Case 58	58
Case 59	59
Case 60	60
Case 61	61
Case 62	62

Case 63   63
Case 64   64
Case 65   65
Case 66   66
Case 67   67
Case 68   68
Case 69   69
Case 70   70
Case 71   71
Case 72   72
Case 73   73
Case 74   74
Case 75   75
Case 76   76

ORTHOPEDIC

Case 77   77
Case 78   78
Case 79   79
Case 80   80
Case 81   81
Case 82   82
Case 83   83
Case 84   84
Case 85   85
Case 86   86

GENERAL SURGERY

Case 87   87
Case 88   88
Case 89   89
Case 90   90
Case 91   91
Case 92   92
Case 93   93
Case 94   94

Case 95   95

Case 96   96

NEONATOLOGY

Case 97   97

Case 98   98

ANSWER KEY   99

Q&AS   101

CONTRIBUTORS

Ashraf Zaman, MBBS
New Delhi, India

Chad Silverberg
Philadelphia College of Osteopathic Medicine, Class of 2004
Resident in Internal Medicine, Cleveland Clinic Foundation
Radiology Resident, Christiana Hospital (From 2005)

Chris Buckle
University of Ottawa, Class of 2005

Joseph Hastings
David Geffen School of Medicine at UCLA/ Class of 2006
UCLA School of Public Health, MPH/ Class of 2006

Kyong Un Chong
Joan C. Edwards School of Medicine, West Virginia, Class of 2005

Kaushik Mukherjee
David Geffen School of Medicine at UCLA, Class of 2005

Michael Kenneth Shindle, MD
Johns Hopkins University School of Medicine, Baltimore, MD, Class of 2004
Intern, Orthopedic Surgery, Hospital for Special Surgery, New York NY

Mustaqeem A Siddiqui, MD
Aga Khan University Medical College, Class of 2002
Resident in Internal Medicine, Mayo Clinic, Rochester MN

Sameer Sheth, PhD
David Geffen School of Medicine at UCLA, Class of 2005

ACKNOWLEDGMENTS

Throughout the production of this book, we have had the support of many friends and colleagues. Special thanks to our support team including Andrea Fellows, Anastasia Anderson, Srishti Gupta, Anu Gupta, Mona Pall, Jonathan Kirsch and Chirag Amin. For prior contributions we thank Gianni Le Nguyen, Tarun Mathur, Alex Grimm, Sonia Santos and Elizabeth Sanders.

For submitting comments, corrections, editing, proofreading, and assistance across all of the vignette titles in all editions, we collectively thank:

Tara Adamovich, Carolyn Alexander, Kris Alden, Henry E. Aryan, Lynman Bacolor, Natalie Barteneva, Dean Bartholomew, Debashish Behera, Sumit Bhatia, Sanjay Bindra, Dave Brinton, Julianne Brown, Alexander Brownie, Tamara Callahan, David Canes, Bryan Casey, Aaron Caughey, Hebert Chen, Jonathan Cheng, Arnold Cheung, Arnold Chin, Simion Chiosea, Yoon Cho, Samuel Chung, Gretchen Conant, Vladimir Coric, Christopher Cosgrove, Ronald Cowan, Karekin R. Cunningham, A. Sean Dalley, Rama Dandamudi, Sunit Das, Ryan Armando Dave, John David, Emmanuel de la Cruz, Robert DeMello, Navneet Dhillon, Sharmila Dissanaike, David Donson, Adolf Etchegaray, Alea Eusebio, Priscilla A. Frase, David Frenz, Kristin Gaumer, Yohannes Gebreegziabher, Anil Gehi, Tony George, L.M. Gotanco, Parul Goyal, Alex Grimm, Rajeev Gupta, Ahmad Halim, Sue Hall, David Hasselbacher, Tamra Heimert, Michelle Higley, Dan Hoit, Eric Jackson, Tim Jackson, Sundar Jayaraman, Pei-Ni Jone, Aarchan Joshi, Rajni K. Jutla, Faiyaz Kapadi, Seth Karp, Aaron S. Kesselheim, Sana Khan, Andrew Pin-wei Ko, Francis Kong, Paul Konitzky, Warren S. Krackov, Benjamin H.S. Lau, Ann LaCasce, Connie Lee, Scott Lee, Guillermo Lehmann, Kevin Leung, Paul Levett, Warren Levinson, Eric Ley, Ken Lin, Pavel Lobanov, J. Mark Maddox, Aram Mardian, Samir Mehta, Gil Melmed, Joe Messina, Robert Mosca, Michael Murphy, Kristen Lem Mygdal, Vivek Nandkarni, Siva Naraynan, Robert Nason, Carvell Nguyen, Hoang Nguyen, Linh Nguyen, Deanna Nobleza, Craig Nodurft, George Noumi, Darin T. Okuda, Adam L. Palance, Paul Pamphrus, Jinha Park, Sonny Patel, Ricardo Pietrobon, Riva L. Rahl, Aashita Randeria, Rachan Reddy, Beatriu Reig, Marilou Reyes, Jeremy Richmon, Tai Roe, Rick Roller, Rajiv Roy, Diego Ruiz, Anthony Russell, Sanjay Sahgal, Urmimala Sarkar, John Schilling, Isabell Schmitt, Daren Schuhmacher, Kalpita Shah, Sonal Shah, Fadi Abu Shahin, Edie Shen, Justin Smith, John Stulak, Lillian Su, Julie Sundaram, Rita Suri, Seth Sweetser, Antonio Talayero, Merita Tan, Mark Tanaka, Eric Taylor, Jess Thompson, Indi Trehan, Raymond Turner, Okafo Uchenna, Eric Uyguanco, Richa Varma, John Wages, Alan Wang, Eunice Wang, Andy Weiss, Amy Williams, Brian Yang, Hany Zaky, Ashraf Zaman and David Zipf.

Please let us know if your name has been missed or misspelled and we will be happy to make the update in the next edition.

For generously contributing images to the entire Underground Clinical Vignette Step 1 series, we collectively thank the staff at Blackwell Publishing in Oxford, Boston, and Berlin as well as:

- Axford, J. Medicine. Osney Mead: Blackwell Science Ltd, 1996. Figures 2.14, 2.15, 2.16, 2.27, 2.28, 2.31, 2.35, 2.36, 2.38, 2.43, 2.65a, 2.65b, 2.65c, 2.103b, 2.105b, 3.20b, 3.21, 8.27, 8.27b, 8.77b, 8.77c, 10.81b, 10.96a, 12.28a, 14.6, 14.16, 14.50.

- Bannister B, Begg N, Gillespie S. Infectious Disease, 2nd Edition. Osney Mead: Blackwell Science Ltd, 2000. Figures 2.8, 3.4, 5.28, 18.10, W5.32, W5.6.

- Berg D. Advanced Clinical Skills and Physical Diagnosis. Blackwell Science Ltd., 1999. Figures 7.10, 7.12, 7.13, 7.2, 7.3, 7.7, 7.8, 7.9, 8.1, 8.2, 8.4, 8.5, 9.2, 10.2, 11.3, 11.5, 12.6.

- Cuschieri A, Hennessy TPJ, Greenhalgh RM, Rowley DA, Grace PA. Clinical Surgery. Osney Mead: Blackwell Science Ltd, 1996. Figures 13.19, 18.22, 18.33.

- Gillespie SH, Bamford K. *Medical Microbiology and Infection at a Glance.* Osney Mead.: Blackwell Science Ltd, 2000, Figures 20, 23.

- Ginsberg L. Lecture Notes on Neurology, 7th Edition. Osney Mead: Blackwell Science Ltd, 1999. Figures 12.3, 18.3, 18.3b.

- Elliott T, Hastings M, Desselberger U. Lecture Notes on Medical Microbiology, 3rd Edition. Osney Mead: Blackwell Science Ltd, 1997. Figures 2, 5, 7, 8, 9, 11, 12, 14, 15, 16, 17, 19, 20, 25, 26, 27, 29, 30, 34, 35, 52.

- Mehta AB, Hoffbrand AV. Haematology at a Glance. Osney Mead: Blackwell Science Ltd, 2000. Figures 22.1, 22.2, 22.3.

HOW TO USE THIS BOOK

This series was originally developed to address the increasing number of clinical vignette questions on medical examinations, including the USMLE Step 1 and Step 2.

Each UCV 1 book uses a series of approximately **100** "**supra-prototypical**" **cases as a way to condense testable facts and associations.** The clinical vignettes in this series are designed to give added emphasis to pathogenesis, epidemiology, management and complications. Although each case tends to present all the signs, symptoms, and diagnostic findings for a particular illness, **patients generally will not present with such a "complete" picture either clinically or on a medical examination.** Cases are not meant to simulate a potential real patient or an exam vignette. **All the boldfaced "buzzwords" are for learning purposes** and are not necessarily expected to be found in any one patient with the disease.

Definitions of selected important terms are placed within the vignettes in (small caps) in parentheses. Other parenthetical remarks often refer to the pathophysiology or mechanism of disease. The format should also help students learn to present cases succinctly during oral "bullet" presentations on clinical rotations. The cases are meant to serve as a condensed review, not as a primary reference. The information provided in this book has been prepared with a great deal of thought and careful research. This book should not, however, be considered as your sole source of information. Corrections, suggestions and submissions of new cases are encouraged and will be acknowledged and incorporated when appropriate in future editions.

We hope that you find the *Blackwell Underground Clinical Vignettes* series informative and useful. We welcome feedback and suggestions you have about this book, or any published by Blackwell Publishing.

Please e-mail us at medfeedback@bos.blackwellpublishing.com.

ABBREVIATIONS

ABGs	arterial blood gases
ABPA	allergic bronchopulmonary aspergillosis
ACA	anticardiolipin antibody
ACE	angiotensin-converting enzyme
ACL	anterior cruciate ligament
ACTH	adrenocorticotropic hormone
AD	adjustment disorder
ADA	adenosine deaminase
ADD	attention deficit disorder
ADH	antidiuretic hormone
ADHD	attention deficit hyperactivity disorder
ADP	adenosine diphosphate
AFO	ankle-foot orthosis
AFP	α-fetoprotein
AIDS	acquired immunodeficiency syndrome
ALL	acute lymphocytic leukemia
ALS	amyotrophic lateral sclerosis
ALT	alanine aminotransferase
AML	acute myelogenous leukemia
ANA	antinuclear antibody
Angio	angiography
AP	anteroposterior
APKD	adult polycystic kidney disease
aPTT	activated partial thromboplastin time
ARDS	adult respiratory distress syndrome
5-ASA	5-aminosalicylic acid
ASCA	antibodies to *Saccharomyces cerevisiae*
ASO	antistreptolysin O
AST	aspartate aminotransferase
ATLL	adult T-cell leukemia/lymphoma
ATPase	adenosine triphosphatase
AV	arteriovenous, atrioventricular
AZT	azidothymidine (zidovudine)
BAL	British antilewisite (dimercaprol)
BCG	bacille Calmette-Guérin
BE	barium enema
BP	blood pressure
BPH	benign prostatic hypertrophy
BUN	blood urea nitrogen
CABG	coronary artery bypass grafting
CAD	coronary artery disease
CaEDTA	calcium edetate
CALLA	common acute lymphoblastic leukemia antigen
cAMP	cyclic adenosine monophosphate
C-ANCA	cytoplasmic antineutrophil cytoplasmic antibody
CBC	complete blood count

CBD	common bile duct
CCU	cardiac care unit
CD	cluster of differentiation
2-CdA	2-chlorodeoxyadenosine
CEA	carcinoembryonic antigen
CFTR	cystic fibrosis transmembrane conductance regulator
cGMP	cyclic guanosine monophosphate
CHF	congestive heart failure
CK	creatine kinase
CK-MB	creatine kinase, MB fraction
CLL	chronic lymphocytic leukemia
CML	chronic myelogenous leukemia
CMV	cytomegalovirus
CN	cranial nerve
CNS	central nervous system
COPD	chronic obstructive pulmonary disease
COX	cyclooxygenase
CP	cerebellopontine
CPAP	continuous positive airway pressure
CPK	creatine phosphokinase
CPPD	calcium pyrophosphate dihydrate
CPR	cardiopulmonary resuscitation
CREST	calcinosis, Raynaud's phenomenon, esophageal involvement, sclerodactyly, telangiectasia (syndrome)
CRP	C-reactive protein
CSF	cerebrospinal fluid
CSOM	chronic suppurative otitis media
CT	cardiac transplant, computed tomography
CVA	cerebrovascular accident
CXR	chest x-ray
d4T	didehydrodeoxythymidine (stavudine)
DCS	decompression sickness
DDH	developmental dysplasia of the hip
ddI	dideoxyinosine (didanosine)
DES	diethylstilbestrol
DEXA	dual-energy x-ray absorptiometry
DHEAS	dehydroepiandrosterone sulfate
DIC	disseminated intravascular coagulation
DIF	direct immunofluorescence
DIP	distal interphalangeal (joint)
DKA	diabetic ketoacidosis
DL_{CO}	diffusing capacity of carbon monoxide
DMSA	2,3-dimercaptosuccinic acid
DNA	deoxyribonucleic acid
DNase	deoxyribonuclease
2,3-DPG	2,3-diphosphoglycerate

dsDNA	double-stranded DNA
DSM	Diagnostic and Statistical Manual
dsRNA	double-stranded RNA
DTP	diphtheria, tetanus, pertussis (vaccine)
DTPA	diethylenetriamine-penta-acetic acid
DTs	delirium tremens
DVT	deep venous thrombosis
EBV	Epstein-Barr virus
ECG	electrocardiography
Echo	echocardiography
ECM	erythema chronicum migrans
ECT	electroconvulsive therapy
EEG	electroencephalography
EF	ejection fraction, elongation factor
EGD	esophagogastroduodenoscopy
EHEC	enterohemorrhagic *E. coli*
EIA	enzyme immunoassay
ELISA	enzyme-linked immunosorbent assay
EM	electron microscopy
EMG	electromyography
ENT	ears, nose, and throat
EPVE	early prosthetic valve endocarditis
ER	emergency room
ERCP	endoscopic retrograde cholangiopancreatography
ERT	estrogen replacement therapy
ESR	erythrocyte sedimentation rate
ETEC	enterotoxigenic *E. coli*
EtOH	ethanol
FAP	familial adenomatous polyposis
FEV$_1$	forced expiratory volume in 1 second
FH	familial hypercholesterolemia
FNA	fine-needle aspiration
FSH	follicle-stimulating hormone
FTA-ABS	fluorescent treponemal antibody absorption test
FVC	forced vital capacity
G6PD	glucose-6-phosphate dehydrogenase
GABA	gamma-aminobutyric acid
GERD	gastroesophageal reflux disease
GFR	glomerular filtration rate
GGT	gamma-glutamyltransferase
GH	growth hormone
GI	gastrointestinal
GnRH	gonadotropin-releasing hormone
GU	genitourinary
GVHD	graft-versus-host disease
HAART	highly active antiretroviral therapy

HAV	hepatitis A virus
Hb	hemoglobin
HbA-1C	hemoglobin A-1C
HBsAg	hepatitis B surface antigen
HBV	hepatitis B virus
hCG	human chorionic gonadotropin
HCO_3	bicarbonate
Hct	hematocrit
HCV	hepatitis C virus
HDL	high-density lipoprotein
HDL-C	high-density lipoprotein-cholesterol
HEENT	head, eyes, ears, nose, and throat (exam)
HELLP	hemolysis, elevated LFTs, low platelets (syndrome)
HFMD	hand, foot, and mouth disease
HGPRT	hypoxanthine-guanine phosphoribosyltransferase
5-HIAA	5-hydroxyindoleacetic acid
HIDA	hepato-iminodiacetic acid (scan)
HIV	human immunodeficiency virus
HLA	human leukocyte antigen
HMG-CoA	hydroxymethylglutaryl-coenzyme A
HMP	hexose monophosphate
HPI	history of present illness
HPV	human papillomavirus
HR	heart rate
HRIG	human rabies immune globulin
HRS	hepatorenal syndrome
HRT	hormone replacement therapy
HSG	hysterosalpingography
HSV	herpes simplex virus
HTLV	human T-cell leukemia virus
HUS	hemolytic-uremic syndrome
HVA	homovanillic acid
ICP	intracranial pressure
ICU	intensive care unit
ID/CC	identification and chief complaint
IDDM	insulin-dependent diabetes mellitus
IFA	immunofluorescent antibody
Ig	immunoglobulin
IGF	insulin-like growth factor
IHSS	idiopathic hypertrophic subaortic stenosis
IM	intramuscular
IMA	inferior mesenteric artery
INH	isoniazid
INR	International Normalized Ratio
IP_3	inositol 1,4,5-triphosphate
IPF	idiopathic pulmonary fibrosis

ITP	idiopathic thrombocytopenic purpura
IUD	intrauterine device
IV	intravenous
IVC	inferior vena cava
IVIG	intravenous immunoglobulin
IVP	intravenous pyelography
JRA	juvenile rheumatoid arthritis
JVP	jugular venous pressure
KOH	potassium hydroxide
KUB	kidney, ureter, bladder
LCM	lymphocytic choriomeningitis
LDH	lactate dehydrogenase
LDL	low-density lipoprotein
LE	lupus erythematosus (cell)
LES	lower esophageal sphincter
LFTs	liver function tests
LH	luteinizing hormone
LMN	lower motor neuron
LP	lumbar puncture
LPVE	late prosthetic valve endocarditis
L/S	lecithin-sphingomyelin (ratio)
LSD	lysergic acid diethylamide
LT	labile toxin
LV	left ventricular
LVH	left ventricular hypertrophy
Lytes	electrolytes
Mammo	mammography
MAO	monoamine oxidase (inhibitor)
MCP	metacarpophalangeal (joint)
MCTD	mixed connective tissue disorder
MCV	mean corpuscular volume
MEN	multiple endocrine neoplasia
MI	myocardial infarction
MIBG	meta-iodobenzylguanidine (radioisotope)
MMR	measles, mumps, rubella (vaccine)
MPGN	membranoproliferative glomerulonephritis
MPS	mucopolysaccharide
MPTP	1-methyl-4-phenyl-tetrahydropyridine
MR	magnetic resonance (imaging)
mRNA	messenger ribonucleic acid
MRSA	methicillin-resistant *S. aureus*
MTP	metatarsophalangeal (joint)
NAD	nicotinamide adenine dinucleotide
NADP	nicotinamide adenine dinucleotide phosphate
NADPH	reduced nicotinamide adenine dinucleotide phosphate
NF	neurofibromatosis

NIDDM	non-insulin-dependent diabetes mellitus
NNRTI	non-nucleoside reverse transcriptase inhibitor
NO	nitric oxide
NPO	nil per os (nothing by mouth)
NSAID	nonsteroidal anti-inflammatory drug
Nuc	nuclear medicine
NYHA	New York Heart Association
OB	obstetric
OCD	obsessive-compulsive disorder
OCPs	oral contraceptive pills
OR	operating room
PA	posteroanterior
PABA	para-aminobenzoic acid
PAN	polyarteritis nodosa
P-ANCA	perinuclear antineutrophil cytoplasmic antibody
Pao_2	partial pressure of oxygen in arterial blood
PAS	periodic acid Schiff
PAT	paroxysmal atrial tachycardia
PBS	peripheral blood smear
Pco_2	partial pressure of carbon dioxide
PCOM	posterior communicating (artery)
PCOS	polycystic ovarian syndrome
PCP	phencyclidine
PCR	polymerase chain reaction
PCT	porphyria cutanea tarda
PCTA	percutaneous coronary transluminal angioplasty
PCV	polycythemia vera
PDA	patent ductus arteriosus
PDGF	platelet-derived growth factor
PE	physical exam
PEFR	peak expiratory flow rate
PEG	polyethylene glycol
PEPCK	phosphoenolpyruvate carboxykinase
PET	positron emission tomography
PFTs	pulmonary function tests
PID	pelvic inflammatory disease
PIP	proximal interphalangeal (joint)
PKU	phenylketonuria
PMDD	premenstrual dysphoric disorder
PML	progressive multifocal leukoencephalopathy
PMN	polymorphonuclear (leukocyte)
PNET	primitive neuroectodermal tumor
PNH	paroxysmal nocturnal hemoglobinuria
Po_2	partial pressure of oxygen
PPD	purified protein derivative (of tuberculosis)
PPH	primary postpartum hemorrhage

PRA	panel reactive antibody
PROM	premature rupture of membranes
PSA	prostate-specific antigen
PSS	progressive systemic sclerosis
PT	prothrombin time
PTH	parathyroid hormone
PTSD	post-traumatic stress disorder
PTT	partial thromboplastin time
PUVA	psoralen ultraviolet A
PVC	premature ventricular contraction
RA	rheumatoid arthritis
RAIU	radioactive iodine uptake
RAST	radioallergosorbent test
RBC	red blood cell
REM	rapid eye movement
RES	reticuloendothelial system
RFFIT	rapid fluorescent focus inhibition test
RFTs	renal function tests
RHD	rheumatic heart disease
RNA	ribonucleic acid
RNP	ribonucleoprotein
RPR	rapid plasma reagin
RR	respiratory rate
RSV	respiratory syncytial virus
RUQ	right upper quadrant
RV	residual volume
Sao$_2$	oxygen saturation in arterial blood
SBFT	small bowel follow-through
SCC	squamous cell carcinoma
SCID	severe combined immunodeficiency
SERM	selective estrogen receptor modulator
SGOT	serum glutamic-oxaloacetic transaminase
SIADH	syndrome of inappropriate antidiuretic hormone
SIDS	sudden infant death syndrome
SLE	systemic lupus erythematosus
SMA	superior mesenteric artery
SSPE	subacute sclerosing panencephalitis
SSRI	selective serotonin reuptake inhibitor
ST	stable toxin
STD	sexually transmitted disease
T2W	T2-weighted (MRI)
T$_3$	triiodothyronine
T$_4$	thyroxine
TAH-BSO	total abdominal hysterectomy–bilateral salpingo-oophorectomy
TB	tuberculosis
TCA	tricyclic antidepressant

TCC	transitional cell carcinoma
TDT	terminal deoxytransferase
TFTs	thyroid function tests
TGF	transforming growth factor
THC	tetrahydrocannabinol
TIA	transient ischemic attack
TLC	total lung capacity
TMP-SMX	trimethoprim-sulfamethoxazole
tPA	tissue plasminogen activator
TP-HA	*Treponema pallidum* hemagglutination assay
TPP	thiamine pyrophosphate
TRAP	tartrate-resistant acid phosphatase
tRNA	transfer ribonucleic acid
TSH	thyroid-stimulating hormone
TSS	toxic shock syndrome
TTP	thrombotic thrombocytopenic purpura
TURP	transurethral resection of the prostate
TXA	thromboxane A
UA	urinalysis
UDCA	ursodeoxycholic acid
UGI	upper GI
UPPP	uvulopalatopharyngoplasty
URI	upper respiratory infection
US	ultrasound
UTI	urinary tract infection
UV	ultraviolet
VDRL	Venereal Disease Research Laboratory
VIN	vulvar intraepithelial neoplasia
VIP	vasoactive intestinal polypeptide
VLDL	very low density lipoprotein
VMA	vanillylmandelic acid
V/Q	ventilation/perfusion (ratio)
VRE	vancomycin-resistant enterococcus
VS	vital signs
VSD	ventricular septal defect
vWF	von Willebrand's factor
VZV	varicella-zoster virus
WAGR	Wilms' tumor, aniridia, genitourinary abnormalities, mental retardation (syndrome)
WBC	white blood cell
WHI	Women's Health Initiative
WPW	Wolff-Parkinson-White syndrome
XR	x-ray
ZN	Ziehl-Neelsen (stain)

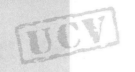
CASE 1

ID/CC   A 48-year-old **male** with a history of **hypertension** is brought by ambulance to the emergency room because of the development of **sudden sharp, tearing, intractable left chest pain with radiation to the back.**

HPI   When he first arrives, he shows a declining level of consciousness, becomes **pale** and **short of breath** (DYSPNEA), has **decreased urine output** (OLIGURIA), and is unable to move his left arm and leg; subsequently he **faints** (SYNCOPE).

PE   VS: **marked hypotension** (BP 90/50) in left arm, with significantly higher reading in right arm (BP 170/80). PE: **pallor; cyanosis; diaphoresis;** indistinct heart sounds; **aortic regurgitation murmur** (high-pitched, blowing, diastolic decrescendo murmur); inspiratory crackles at lung bases bilaterally (due to pulmonary edema); **anuria** (due to decreased renal perfusion); **left-sided hemiplegia.**

Labs   ECG: no evidence of myocardial infarct.

Imaging   CT/MR: **spiraling intimal flap with true and false lumen** (DOUBLE-BARREL AORTA). Angio, aortography: confirmatory. CXR: **mediastinal widening** (due to hemorrhage).

Gross Pathology   Longitudinal separation of tunica media of aortic wall.

Treatment   ICU monitoring for shock; antihypertensive agents (preferably beta-blockers) to decrease vascular shear forces (avoid arteriolar dilators such as hydralazine); surgical correction.

Discussion   Aortic dissection is a **life-threatening** condition requiring immediate treatment. Predisposing factors include **hypertension** and connective tissue diseases (cystic medial degeneration as in Marfan's syndrome); complications include rupture and extension. **Sudden death** may occur with **pericardial tamponade** or **extension of dissection into coronary arteries.**

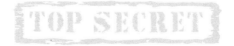

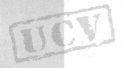
ID/CC	A 31-year-old white male who was diagnosed with **Marfan's syndrome** more than 20 years ago **recently** developed **severe shortness of breath**.
HPI	He denies smoking or drinking and claims to have had no major illnesses in the past.
PE	VS: **pulse bounding, large in volume, and collapsing** (WATER-HAMMER OR CORRIGAN'S PULSE), producing **wide pulse pressure** with rapid rise and fall. PE: soft, high-pitched, blowing **diastolic decrescendo murmur heard best at left sternal border** with patient leaning forward and in expiration; diastolic murmur heard when femoral artery compressed with stethoscope (DUROZIEZ' SIGN).
Labs	ECG: left ventricular hypertrophy (LVH).
Imaging	CXR: left ventricular dilatation. Echo: LVH; Doppler confirmatory.
Gross Pathology	Caused by defect of aortic valves or roots that leads to regurgitation of blood from aorta into left ventricle.
Treatment	Surgical **prosthetic valve replacement** for symptomatic patients or for asymptomatic patients with LV dysfunction. For symptomatic patients with normal LV function, diuretics or afterload-reducing drugs may be beneficial. Antibiotic prophylaxis against infective endocarditis before undergoing surgical or dental procedures.
Discussion	Common causes of aortic insufficiency include congenital bicuspid valve and infective endocarditis; less common causes include rheumatic heart disease and aortic root diseases (e.g., Marfan's syndrome, ankylosing spondylitis, Reiter's syndrome, tertiary syphilis).

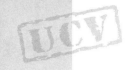

CASE 3

ID/CC A 24-year-old man complains of easy fatigability, dyspnea on mild exertion, and **angina**.

HPI He also admits to having occasional spells of **lightheadedness** and **fainting** while playing basketball.

PE **Crescendo-decrescendo systolic ejection murmur to right of sternum and radiating to neck**; soft S2 with **paradoxical splitting** (due to pulmonary valve closure preceding aortic valve closure); weak and delayed ("parvus et tardus") carotid pulses.

Labs ECG: left ventricular hypertrophy.

Imaging CXR: calcifications on valve leaflets and enlarged cardiac shadow (due to large left ventricle). Echo: presence of bicuspid aortic valve.

Gross Pathology Congenital bicuspid valve with calcification.

Treatment Balloon valvuloplasty; surgical aortic valve replacement; antibiotic prophylaxis with penicillin prior to surgical or dental procedures.

Discussion Causes of aortic stenosis include congenital bicuspid aortic valve (more common in males), progressive degenerative calcification of normal valves (more common in elderly males), and rheumatic heart disease (the mitral valve is also involved in 95% of individuals with rheumatic disease of the aortic valve).

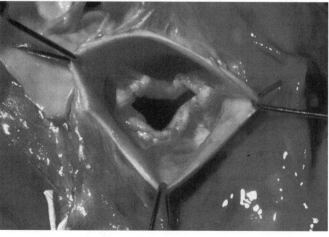

Figure 003 Deformation and calcium deposition of the aortic valve cusps.

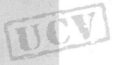

CASE 4

ID/CC   A 59-year-old white male complains of **pain in the calf muscles** during exercise (CLAUDICATION) along with coldness and numbness in both legs; his symptoms have been occurring for a year and are **relieved by rest**.

HPI   The patient has also been **impotent** and has been experiencing abdominal pain (due to mesenteric ischemia) about half an hour after eating (POSTPRANDIAL PAIN). He **smokes** two packs of cigarettes a day.

PE   VS: hypertension (BP 150/100). PE: **diminished peripheral pulses** bilaterally; **loss of hair** over dorsum of feet and hands; decreased temperature in hands and feet; **carotid and femoral arterial bruits**; atrophy of calf muscles.

Labs   Elevated LDL and decreased HDL; elevated total serum cholesterol.

Imaging   Angio: multiple large **atheromatous plaques in aortoiliac distribution**. XR, plain: irregular arterial vascular calcifications. US, Doppler: high-velocity poststenotic flow jet.

Gross Pathology   Early: fatty streak in subendothelium; late: **fibrofatty plaque** formation with dystrophic calcification (atheroma) with narrowing of lumen of vessel wall.

Micro Pathology   Early: **foam cells** with intimal proliferation of smooth muscle cells; late: smooth muscle cells synthesize collagen and form **fibrous cap** with **necrotic lipid core** and fibrous plaque.

Treatment   Exercise; dietary modifications; smoking cessation; low-dose aspirin; control of hypertension; cholesterol-lowering drugs (e.g., lovastatin); angioplasty; coronary stenting; coronary artery bypass grafting (CABG).

Discussion   Atherosclerosis is the main cause of coronary artery disease and the leading cause of mortality in the United States. Plaques are commonly found in the abdominal aorta, coronary arteries, popliteal arteries, descending thoracic aorta, internal carotid arteries, and circle of Willis arteries. Thus, they are responsible for aortic aneurysms, CAD, peripheral vascular disease, intestinal angina, renovascular hypertension, and cerebrovascular disease.

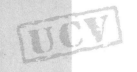

CASE 5

CARDIOLOGY

ID/CC

A 47-year-old man complains of occasional **palpitations** and **shortness of breath**.

HPI

He also says that he occasionally experiences mild **dizziness** and chest discomfort.

PE

VS: **irregularly irregular** pulse. PE: loss of a waves in jugular venous pulse; variable-intensity S1 with occasional S3.

Labs

ECG: variable ventricular rate (80 to 200); can be > 200 with wide QRS if associated with accessory pathway; **no discernible P waves seen**. Normal CK-MB.

Imaging

CXR: normal. Echo: enlarged left atrium.

Treatment

Beta-blockers; calcium channel blockers; digitalis (to decrease conduction at AV node in order to control ventricular rate; chemical cardioversion with **class IA, IC, or III antiarrhythmics** to convert back to sinus rhythm if patient remains symptomatic; **electrical cardioversion**; patients should also be **anticoagulated** with warfarin to prevent embolic disease.

Discussion

Atrial fibrillation, the most common chronic arrhythmia, is associated with a high risk of **embolic disease**. Causes include drugs, mitral valve disease, hypertensive and ischemic heart disease, dilated cardiomyopathy, alcoholism, **hyperthyroidism**, pericarditis, pulmonary embolism, exercise, atrial septal defect, chronic lung disease, and cardiac surgery. It may also be idiopathic.

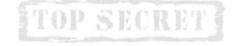

5

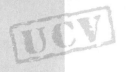

ID/CC

A 50-year-old woman complains of recurrent, transient losses of consciousness (SYNCOPE) and dizziness.

HPI

For the past few months she has had continuous mild to moderate fever, fatigue, sweating, and joint pains (ARTHRALGIAS) and has experienced unexplainable breathlessness at rest (episodic pulmonary edema) that is relieved in a supine position and exacerbated by standing. She also complains of significant weight loss over the past year.

PE

VS: mild fever. PE: pallor and clubbing; on auscultation, S1 delayed and decreased in intensity and characteristic low-pitched sound (tumor plop) during early diastole, followed by a rumble; auscultatory findings vary with body position.

Labs

CBC: normochromic, normocytic anemia. Elevated ESR; increased IgG; blood cultures sterile. ECG: sinus rhythm.

Imaging

Echo (2D): characteristic echo-producing mass in left atrium. MR, cardiac: globular mass in left atrium.

Gross Pathology

Single globular left atrial mass about 6 cm in diameter, pedunculated with fibrovascular stalk arising from interatrial septum in vicinity of fossa ovalis (favored site of atrial origin).

Micro Pathology

Stellate, multipotential mesenchymal myxoma cells mixed with endothelial cells; mature and immature smooth muscle cells and macrophages, all in an acid mucopolysaccharide matrix.

Treatment

Surgical excision using cardiopulmonary bypass is curative.

Discussion

The most common type of primary cardiac tumors, myxomas may be located in any of the four chambers or, rarely, in the valves. They are predominantly atrial with a 4:1 left-to-right ratio and are usually single. Their signs and symptoms are closely related to their location and to the patient's position. Although myxomas are benign, they can embolize, resulting in metastatic disease. Although most myxomas are sporadic, some are familial with autosomal-dominant transmission; thus, echocardiographic screening of first-degree relatives is appropriate.

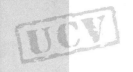

ID/CC

A **78-year-old** white **male** is brought into the emergency room with **nausea, dyspnea**, and a **crushing substernal chest pain** that radiates to his **left arm and jaw**; the pain has lasted for about 30 minutes and is not relieved with rest.

HPI

One sublingual nitroglycerin tablet did not relieve his pain. His history reveals a **sedentary lifestyle, moderate hypercholesterolemia**, and obesity. The patient is also a **diabetic** and **smokes**.

PE

VS: hypotension. PE: **diaphoresis**.

Labs

ECG: **ST elevation** with peaking of T waves; subsequent development of **inverted T waves** and **permanent Q waves**. Later, ST and T waves normalize. **Elevated CK-MB; elevated troponin T and I**. CBC: leukocytosis.

Imaging

Echo: **decreased wall motion** (HYPOKINESIS).

Gross Pathology

12 hours: no myocardial damage; 24 hours: pallor due to coagulation necrosis or reddish mottling; 3 to 5 days: demarcated yellow region with hyperemic border; 2 to 3 weeks: soft, gelatinous; 1 to 2 months: white scar and firm, thin wall.

Micro Pathology

12 to 18 hours: nuclear pyknosis, **coagulation necrosis**, and eosinophilia; 1 to 3 days: intense neutrophilic infiltrate, loss of nuclei and cross-striations; 1 week: disappearance of PMNs, onset of fibroblastic repair; 3 weeks: granulation tissue with progressive fibrosis.

Treatment

Oxygen, bed rest, aspirin, pain relief with morphine, nitrates, beta-blockers; plaque stabilization with heparin, anti-Gp IIa-IIIb monoclonal antibodies; thrombolysis with tPA if cardiac catheterization is not immediately available; cardiac catheterization with angioplasty or surgical reperfusion with a bypass graft depending on nature of disease; ACE inhibitors (limit postinfarct remodeling) and cholesterol-lowering drugs.

Discussion

The most common cause of myocardial infarction is atherosclerosis (coronary artery disease); it is less commonly caused by coronary vasospasm (Prinzmetal's angina). Sequelae include arrhythmias, congestive heart failure, pulmonary edema, shock, pulmonary embolism, papillary muscle rupture, ventricular aneurysm, ventricular wall rupture, tamponade, and autoimmune fibrinous pericarditis (DRESSLER'S SYNDROME).

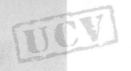

ID/CC   A 50-year-old male who was admitted to the CCU **3 days ago** following an **MI** presents with **hypotension**.

HPI   The patient was thrombolyzed post-MI and was recovering well. He also complained of a mild fever but no chills or rigors.

PE   VS: tachycardia; weak, thready pulse; tachypnea; **hypotension**. PE: pallor; cool, moist skin; mild cyanosis of lips and digits; > 10-mmHg fall in arterial pressure with inspiration (PULSUS PARADOXUS); **heart sounds muffled** and **JVP elevated**; lungs clear bilaterally.

Labs   Elevated cardiac enzymes (CK-MB, troponin) as a result of recent acute MI.

Imaging   Echo: diastolic compression of the right ventricle; pericardial effusion.

Gross Pathology   Rupture of the left ventricular wall with hemopericardium.

Micro Pathology   Ischemic coagulative necrosis of the affected myocardium, consisting of multiple erythrocytes and dead, anucleated myocytes.

Treatment   Emergency pericardiocentesis; treat shock by infusing fluid and isoproterenol; surgical repair of cardiac rupture subsequent to stabilization.

Discussion   Cardiac rupture most typically develops 3 to 10 days after the initial onset of the infarction secondary to rupture of necrotic cardiac muscle; there is usually little warning before the sudden collapse, which is associated with acute cardiac tamponade and electromechanical dissociation. Papillary muscle rupture may also occur following an acute MI, resulting in mitral regurgitation and left ventricular failure.

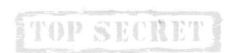

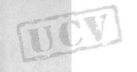

CASE 9

CARDIOLOGY

ID/CC

A 60-year-old male presents to a clinic for a **heart transplant evaluation**.

HPI

The patient was diagnosed last year with **class III** (marked limitation of activity; comfortable only at rest) **congestive heart failure** secondary to **idiopathic dilated cardiomyopathy**. He is currently being treated with digoxin, furosemide (diuretic), lisinopril (ACE inhibitor), and warfarin (anticoagulant) but continues to be symptomatic.

PE

VS: normal. PE: elevated JVP; S3/S4 gallop heard on auscultation; significant pitting lower extremity **edema**.

Labs

CBC/Lytes: Normal. TFTs, LFTs, total protein, albumin, uric acid, and 24-hour protein/creatinine normal; PSA normal; IgG and IgM antibody titers against CMV, HSV, HIV, VZV, hepatitis B and C, and toxoplasmosis negative; PT/PTT/INR normal.

Imaging

Echo: EF 15% with moderate mitral valve regurgitation. CXR: **cardiomegaly**. ECG: occasional **premature ventricular contractions (PVCs)**. Thallium scan: **exercise-induced global cardiac ischemia**.

Treatment

If approved as a viable transplant candidate, the patient must wait for a suitable donor (matched according to body size, weight, **ABO blood grouping**, and levels of **panel reactive antibody, or PRA**). A large number of patients waiting for a cardiac transplant (CT) die before a donor can be found.

Discussion

Cardiac transplantation accounts for 14% of organ transplant procedures and can dramatically improve cardiac function in individuals with end-stage cardiac disease. Patients must have **New York Heart Association (NYHA) class III or IV congestive heart failure**, having failed maximum medical therapy and other therapeutic interventions such as PCTA for CAD. Currently, **ischemic heart disease** accounts for approximately 55% of causes requiring CT and **idiopathic cardiomyopathy** for roughly 40%.

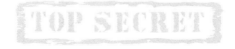

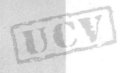

ID/CC
A 65-year-old white male complains of **requiring three pillows in bed in order to breathe comfortably** (ORTHOPNEA) and having to open the window to **gasp for air at night** (PAROXYSMAL NOCTURNAL DYSPNEA).

HPI
He has also noted **increasing shortness of breath** while walking as well as **swelling of his ankles and legs**. He had a **myocardial infarction** 2 years ago and has a history of **chronic hypertension**.

PE
VS: tachycardia; tachypnea; weak, thready pulse. PE: central cyanosis; **distention of neck veins** (due to elevated JVP); **third heart sound**; grade III/VI crescendo aortic systolic murmur; **crepitant rales** over both lower lobes; **lower lung fields dull to percussion** bilaterally; tender hepatomegaly; **4+ pitting edema** in both lower extremities; cold extremities.

Labs
ABGs: hypoxemia; **low cardiac output** as measured by Fick equation and Swan-Ganz catheter (2.4 L/min); transudate in pleural fluid; increased BUN. ECG: left ventricular hypertrophy.

Imaging
CXR: enlarged cardiac silhouette; bilateral pleural effusions and diffuse increased lung markings (KERLEY B LINES) suggesting pulmonary edema. Echo: **ejection fraction of 40%**.

Gross Pathology
Cardiomegaly due to both dilatation and hypertrophy; pulmonary edema with increase in weight and reddish-purple color; **nutmeg liver** (due to chronic passive congestion).

Micro Pathology
Hepatization of lungs with alveolar capillary congestion and alveolar macrophages with hemosiderin ("HEART FAILURE CELLS"); centrilobular liver congestion.

Treatment
Diuretics; low-sodium diet, digoxin; ACE inhibitors; nitrates; anti-arrhythmics.

Discussion
Congestive heart failure (CHF) is heart failure due to a deficit in myocardial strength or to an increase in workload. CHF is a common complication of ischemic and hypertensive heart disease in older populations.

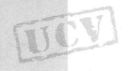

CASE 11

ID/CC   A 35-year-old female **Asian** immigrant complains of weakness, **shortness of breath on exertion**, and **swelling of both feet**.

HPI   She also complains of **progressive abdominal distention** and fatigue. She was treated for **pulmonary tuberculosis** a few years ago.

PE   VS: mild hypotension; **reduced pulse pressure**. PE: peripheral cyanosis and cold extremities; pallor; neck veins distended; **JVP increases during inspiration** (KUSSMAUL'S SIGN); pedal edema; moderate hepatomegaly, splenomegaly, and ascites; **reduced-intensity apical impulse, distant heart sounds, and early third heart sound (pericardial knock)**; no pulsus paradoxus; no murmur or rub heard.

Labs   ECG: **low-voltage** QRS complexes with flattening of T wave (nonspecific). LFTs mildly abnormal (due to hepatic congestion); ascitic fluid **transudative** (low protein, high sugar). UA: proteinuria, no casts.

Imaging   CXR: **fibrosis** (old healed tuberculosis); heart shadow shows signs of **pericardial calcification**. Echo: **pericardial thickening**; dilated IVC and hepatic veins with absent collapse. MR: pericardial **calcification** and **thickening**; dilated IVC.

Gross Pathology   Thick, dense, **fibrous obliteration of pericardial space with calcification** encasing the heart and **limiting diastolic filling**.

Treatment   **Complete pericardial resection** is the only definitive treatment; institute **antituberculous therapy** when appropriate; diuretics; sodium restriction; digitalis for associated atrial fibrillation (in one-third of patients).

Discussion   The etiology of constrictive pericarditis lies in the formation of scar tissue that encases the heart and interferes with ventricular filling. **Tuberculosis** is the most common cause worldwide. Most cases now seen in the United States are idiopathic, but cases resulting from exposure to radiation, trauma, cardiac surgery, rheumatoid arthritis, or uremia have become more common.

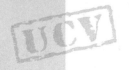

ID/CC   A 60-year-old white male who has been treated for **COPD** comes to the emergency room with severe **dyspnea at rest**.

HPI   Over the past few months, the patient has noted an **increased productive cough** and **exertional dyspnea**. He admits to being a **heavy smoker** and failed to quit smoking even after the appearance of **symptoms and the diagnosis of COPD**.

PE   **Elevated JVP** with large a and v waves; **loud P2**; cyanosis; bilateral wheezing; expiratory rhonchi; prolonged expiration; use of accessory muscles of respiration; left parasternal heave; **ankle and sacral edema**; tender hepatomegaly.

Labs   ECG: **right-axis deviation** and **peaked P waves** (P PULMONALE). PFTs: COPD pattern.

Imaging   CXR: right ventricular and **pulmonary artery enlargement; hyper-inflation**.

Gross Pathology   Right ventricular hypertrophy.

Treatment   Oxygen; salt and water restriction; treatment of COPD.

Discussion   **Cor pulmonale** is **right heart failure due to a pulmonary cause**, most commonly COPD. Other causes are pulmonary fibrosis, pneumoconioses, recurrent pulmonary embolism, primary pulmonary hypertension, obesity with sleep apnea, cystic fibrosis, bronchiectasis, and kyphoscoliosis.

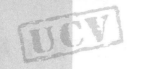

ID/CC	A 29-year-old female who **recently gave birth** to a healthy infant develops **dyspnea** and **swelling of her feet** toward the end of the day.
HPI	She is nursing her 6-week-old child.
PE	VS: BP mildly elevated. PE: JVP raised with prominent a and v waves; tender, mild hepatosplenomegaly; cardiac apex heaving and displaced outside midclavicular line; **pansystolic apical murmur** (due to **mitral insufficiency**) and systolic murmur increasing with inspiration heard in tricuspid area (due to tricuspid insufficiency); loud pulmonary component of S2; S3 and S4 gallop; fine inspiratory basal crepitant rales at both lung bases; pedal edema.
Labs	ECG: premature ventricular contractions.
Imaging	CXR: interstitial pulmonary edema (due to severe pulmonary venous hypertension); **global cardiomegaly**. Echo/Nuc: cardiomegaly with diminished ventricular contractility (**systolic dysfunction**). Stress test: **decreased ejection fraction with stress** (ejection fraction normally increases with stress).
Gross Pathology	Global dilatation of all chambers.
Micro Pathology	**Extensive fibrosis without active inflammation** on endocardial biopsy.
Treatment	Treat cardiac failure with salt restriction, diuretics, vasodilators such as hydralazine (in pregnant patients) or ACE inhibitors (in nonpregnant patients), and digoxin; chronic **anticoagulation**; nutritional supplementation; consider cardiac transplant if medical therapy fails.
Discussion	Dilated cardiomyopathy may develop in the **peripartum period** (± 3 months). Other etiologies include **ischemic heart disease, alcoholism** (due to thiamine deficiency or direct toxicity), hypothyroidism, Friedreich's ataxia, previous **myocarditis** (usually due to **coxsackie B**), myotonic dystrophy, chronic hypocalcemia or hypophosphatemia, **sarcoidosis**, and drug toxicities (e.g., **adriamycin**, cyclophosphamide, **tricyclic antidepressants, lithium**, and cobalt).

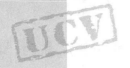

ID/CC   A 23-year-old woman is seen with complaints of **excessive breathlessness, palpitations, fatigue, blood-streaked sputum** (MILD HEMOPTYSIS), **and swelling of the feet** (EDEMA).

HPI   She was diagnosed with **ventricular septal defect** (VSD) at birth, but her parents had refused surgery.

PE   VS: HR, BP normal; mild tachypnea; no fever. PE: **central cyanosis**; clubbing; JVP normal; left parasternal heave; P2 palpable; single second heart sound, predominantly loud P2 (due to pulmonary hypertension); pansystolic murmur along left sternal edge; ejection systolic murmur in pulmonary area; **mid-diastolic murmur** (GRAHAM STEELL MURMUR OF PULMONARY REGURGITATION) **in pulmonary area that increased with inspiration** (CARVALLO'S SIGN, INDICATING RIGHT-SIDED MURMUR).

Labs   ABGs: hypercapnia, hypoxia, and partly compensated respiratory acidosis. CBC: **polycythemia**. ECG: **right ventricular hypertrophy** with right-axis deviation. Cardiac catheterization reveals right-to-left shunt, **pulmonary arterial hypertension**, and pulmonary regurgitation.

Imaging   Echo (with Doppler): **VSD with right-to-left systolic shunt**; right ventricular enlargement and hypertrophy. CXR: pulmonary oligemia ("peripheral pruning") and greatly enlarged hilar pulmonary artery shadows; cardiomegaly.

Treatment   Heart-lung transplantation; surgical correction of a VSD is ideally performed before irreversible pulmonary vascular changes set in.

Discussion   The term "Eisenmenger's syndrome" applies to those defects in which pulmonary vascular disease causes right-to-left shunt of blood; Eisenmenger's complex is right-to-left shunt due to a large VSD. The risk of infective endocarditis is high; therefore, antimicrobial prophylaxis is mandatory. Pregnancy is contraindicated owing to a high maternal mortality rate.

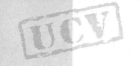

CASE 15

ID/CC

A 20-year-old college student is brought back from a summer camp in the mountains after developing **severe shortness of breath** (DYSPNEA), cough with **blood-tinged sputum** (HEMOPTYSIS), and wheezing.

HPI

The group had **ascended to a height** of 8,000 feet and had engaged in **strenuous physical activities**. The patient subsequently developed dyspnea and cough that worsened during the night, leading to **marked respiratory distress and a shock-like state**.

PE

VS: tachycardia; tachypnea; hypotension. PE: **central cyanosis**; pale and cold extremities; marked **respiratory distress**; **widespread rales and rhonchi** over both lung fields.

Labs

CBC: **elevated hematocrit and hemoglobin**; mildly increased WBC. ABGs: markedly **decreased arterial Po_2** (hypoxia); **low Pco_2. Increased pH** (respiratory alkalosis). ECG: sinus tachycardia.

Imaging

CXR (PA view): **noncardiogenic pulmonary edema** and prominent main pulmonary artery.

Micro Pathology

Extensive pulmonary edema; protein-rich exudate with alveolar hemorrhages and **alveolar hyaline membranes**.

Treatment

Prompt descent, hyperbaric oxygen inhalation, sublingual nifedipine (after checking blood pressure), inhaled nitric oxide, and placement in portable hyperbaric chamber while being transported; hospital management consists of **continuous high-flow oxygen, dexamethasone for CNS symptoms, and acetazolamide**.

Discussion

High-altitude pulmonary edema is primarily a disorder of the pulmonary circulation **induced by sustained alveolar hypoxia**. The initiating event is an abnormal degree of **hypoxia-induced pulmonary arteriolar (precapillary) constriction** (hypoxia causes dilatation of systemic blood vessels) that elevates pulmonary arterial pressure. The imbalance of **increased blood flow** and pressure allows fluid to leave the pulmonary vasculature, resulting in **edema**.

high - altitude sickness

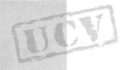

CASE 16

ID/CC A 21-year-old white male presents with anginal chest pain, **dyspnea on exertion**, and an episode of **syncope while playing basketball.**

HPI The patient has no history of blue spells, squatting for relief, or rheumatic fever in childhood.

PE VS: pulse bisferious (DOUBLE PEAKED). PE: JVP normal; cardiac apex forceful with strong presystolic impulse (DOUBLE APICAL IMPULSE); systolic thrill palpable over left sternal border; S4; **ejection systolic murmur** over left third intercostal space radiating to base and axilla; murmur **increased by exercise and during forced expiration against a closed glottis** (VALSALVA MANEUVER) but **decreased by squatting.**

Labs ECG: left-axis deviation due to **left ventricular hypertrophy**; Q wave exaggerated in inferior and lateral precordial leads (due to septal hypertrophy).

Imaging CXR, PA: often normal. Echo: **asymmetrical septal hypertrophy and systolic anterior motion of mitral valve**; Doppler may show **mitral regurgitation**. Angio, cardiac: marked **thickening of left ventricular septal wall**; small ventricular cavity with impaired ventricular filling (diastolic dysfunction) and narrow outflow tract ("HOURGLASS" APPEARANCE).

Gross Pathology Enlarged heart with increased weight and **asymmetrical septal hypertrophy.**

Micro Pathology Myocyte disarray with increased norepinephrine content.

Treatment Negative inotropic agents (e.g., **beta-blockers**, calcium channel blockers) to decrease stiffness of left ventricle and prevent fatal arrhythmias; **avoidance of competitive sports**; surgical myomectomy of interventricular septum in patients with outflow obstruction.

Discussion Also known as **idiopathic hypertrophic subaortic stenosis (IHSS)**. An **autosomal-dominant** pattern of disease is noted in 50% of cases; ventricular outflow tract obstruction by hypertrophy produces symptoms. The presenting symptom in **athletes** might be **sudden death** secondary to lethal cardiac arrhythmias.

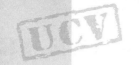

ID/CC

A 28-year-old woman **found on a park bench apparently dead** is brought to the ER in the early hours of the morning.

HPI

No discernible pulse was palpated, but a **faint, infrequent respiratory effort was noted**; CPR was begun and continued during her transport to the hospital. The **temperature overnight was near-freezing** with continuous rain.

PE

VS: arterial **pulse not palpated**; hypotension; reduced respiratory rate; **severe hypothermia (< 28°C)**. PE: no respiratory effort; **fixed and dilated pupils**; blotchy areas of erythema on skin; bullae over buttocks; chest exam shows diffuse rales bilaterally; absent bowel sounds; absent deep tendon reflexes.

Labs

CBC: increased hematocrit. Hypoglycemia; increased BUN and creatinine. Lytes: decreased bicarbonate; hyperkalemia. ABGs: severe metabolic acidosis. ECG: evidence of **marked bradycardia** with **J (Osborn) waves** (upward waves immediately following the S wave).

Imaging

CXR: patchy atelectasis.

Treatment

Intubation and ventilation as necessary; cardiac massage for arrest; warm the patient through use of a combination of heated blankets, heat packs, warm gastric lavage, warm-water immersion, and high-flow oxygen; monitor cardiac rhythm for arrhythmias.

Discussion

Hypothermia is defined as core temperature below 35°C; **severe accidental hypothermia (below 30°C, or 86°F) is associated with marked depression in cerebral blood flow and cerebral oxygen requirement, reduced cardiac output, and decreased arterial pressure.** Victims can **appear to be lifeless** as a result of marked depression of brain function. Peripheral pulses may be difficult to detect because of bradycardia and vasoconstriction. Complications of systemic hypothermia may include ventricular fibrillation, pancreatitis, renal failure, and coagulopathy.

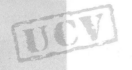

CASE 18

ID/CC	A 42-year-old black male presents with **chest pain, headache, altered mental status, and confusion.**
HPI	He is known to have **labile essential hypertension.** He has no history of fever.
PE	VS: **severe diastolic hypertension** (BP 230/150). PE: **disoriented and confused; bilateral papilledema**; no focal neurologic deficits; remainder of exam normal.
Labs	CBC: microangiopathic hemolytic anemia. UA: **hematuria** and **proteinuria. Increased BUN and serum creatinine.** ECG: **left ventricular hypertrophy.**
Imaging	CT/US, abdomen: bilateral **small and scarred kidneys.**
Gross Pathology	Kidney surface appears "**flea-bitten**" (due to rupture of cortical arterioles and glomerular capillaries).
Micro Pathology	Renal biopsy (not routinely indicated) shows **hyperplastic arteriolosclerosis** ("ONION SKINNING") of interlobular arteries with **fibrinoid necrosis** and thrombi in arterioles and small arteries; **necrotizing glomerulitis** with neutrophil infiltration also seen.
Treatment	Emergent control of hypertension with IV nitroprusside, labetalol, or metoprolol followed by aggressive blood pressure control with oral medications.
Discussion	**End-organ damage** caused by malignant hypertension includes hemorrhagic and lacunar strokes, encephalopathy, fundal hemorrhages, papilledema, myocardial ischemia/infarction, left ventricular hypertrophy, congestive heart failure, acute renal failure, nephrosclerosis, aortic dissection, and necrotizing vasculitis.

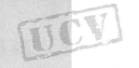
CASE 19

ID/CC The case of a 50-year-old man who died of bleeding complications is discussed at an autopsy meeting owing to **peculiar vegetations seen on his mitral valve**.

HPI He underwent surgery for **adenocarcinoma of the stomach**. Shortly before his death he was diagnosed as having **disseminated intravascular coagulation (DIC)**; he subsequently died of bleeding complications.

Gross Pathology Small (1- to 5-mm) **friable, sterile vegetations** loosely adherent to **mitral valve leaflets along lines of closure**.

Micro Pathology Vegetations found to be **sterile fibrin and platelet thrombi** loosely attached **without evidence of inflammation** (bland) or valve damage.

Discussion Nonbacterial thrombotic endocarditis characteristically occurs in settings of **prolonged debilitating diseases** such as cancer (particularly visceral adenocarcinomas), DIC, renal failure, chronic sepsis, or other **hypercoagulable states**. The vegetations may produce emboli and subsequent infarctions in the heart, kidneys, brain, mesentery, or extremities.

marantic endocarditis

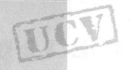

CASE 20

ID/CC	A 37-year-old white male complains of increasing **fatigue** and shortness of breath **during minimal physical exertion**.
HPI	He denies having had any chest pain or having any previous history of similar symptoms. A careful history reveals **rheumatic fever** at age 7.
PE	VS: jerky pulse (RAPID UPSTROKE). PE: high-pitched **pansystolic murmur at apex with radiation to axilla**; S3.
Labs	ECG: left-axis deviation; left atrial and left ventricular hypertrophy.
Imaging	CXR/Echo: enlargement of left atrium and ventricle. Doppler: confirmatory.
Treatment	Oral arteriolar vasodilators (e.g., ACE inhibitors, hydralazine) to improve forward cardiac output; surgical repair or prosthetic replacement; antibiotic prophylaxis with penicillin prior to surgical or dental procedures.
Discussion	Common causes of mitral insufficiency include **mitral valve prolapse**, ischemic papillary muscle dysfunction, infective endocarditis, hypertrophic cardiomyopathy, ventricular enlargement, mitral annulus calcification, and dilated cardiomyopathy; rheumatic heart disease is no longer the leading cause.

TOP SECRET

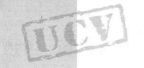

ID/CC
A 34-year-old white female in her 27th week of pregnancy is admitted to the hospital with **dyspnea** and **orthopnea**.

HPI
The patient denies any prior cardiovascular disease, but a careful history reveals that she suffered from **streptococcal pharyngitis** and **rheumatic heart disease** as a child.

PE
Malar flush; elevated JVP (due to venous congestion); left parasternal heave; loud S1; **opening snap**; rumbling, low-pitched **mid-diastolic murmur** at **apex** heard best in left lateral position.

Labs
ECG: **left atrial hypertrophy** and/or **atrial fibrillation**.

Imaging
CXR: double silhouette due to enlarged left atrium; Kerley B lines (due to interstitial edema). Echo: **leaflet thickening** with **fusion of the commissures**.

Gross Pathology
Thickened and scarred mitral valve.

Treatment
Diuretics to relieve pulmonary congestion; treatment of concomitant atrial fibrillation with ventricular rate control (using digoxin) and anticoagulation; valvuloplasty or prosthetic valve replacement; antibiotic prophylaxis against infective endocarditis prior to surgical or dental procedures.

Discussion
The most common cause of mitral stenosis is rheumatic heart disease. The main changes to the valve include leaflet thickening, fusion of the commissures, and shortening, thickening, and fusion of the cordae tendineae.

TOP SECRET

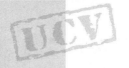

CASE 22

ID/CC
An 18-year-old white **male** complains of gradually progressing **shortness of breath** and **ankle swelling**.

HPI
His symptoms started following a URI. He also complains of **excessive fatigue and frequent chest pain**. He has no history of joint pain, skin rash, or involuntary movements (vs. rheumatic fever) and is neither hypertensive nor diabetic.

PE
VS: tachycardia; hypotension; no fever. PE: **elevated JVP**; pitting pedal edema; fine inspiratory rales at both lung bases; mild tender hepatomegaly; splenomegaly; **right-sided S3**; murmurs of mitral regurgitation.

Labs
ASO titers not raised. CBC: lymphocytosis. Elevated ESR. ECG: **first-degree AV block with nonspecific ST-T changes**. **Coxsackievirus** isolated on pharyngeal washings; increased titers of serum antibodies to coxsackievirus; **elevated cardiac enzymes**.

Imaging
CXR: cardiomegaly and pulmonary edema. Echo: suggestive of dilated cardiomyopathy with low ejection fraction.

Gross Pathology
Flabby, dilated heart with foci of myocardial petechial hemorrhages.

Micro Pathology
Endomyocardial biopsy reveals **diffuse infiltration by mononuclear cells, predominantly lymphocytes**; interstitial edema; focal myofiber necrosis; focal fibrosis.

Treatment
Rest; specific antimicrobial therapy when appropriate; control of congestive cardiac failure by diuretics, digitalis, and vasodilators; antiarrhythmics if indicated; cardiac transplant in intractable cases. Although most cases of acute myocarditis may resolve spontaneously, some progress to dilated cardiomyopathy.

Discussion
The etiology of myocarditis is usually coxsackie B or other viruses; less often implicated are bacteria or fungi, rickettsiae (e.g., Rocky Mountain spotted fever), spirochetes (e.g., Lyme disease), *Trypanosoma cruzi* (Chagas' disease), hypersensitivity disease (SLE, drug reaction), radiation, and sarcoidosis. Diphtheria toxin also causes myocarditis by inhibiting eukaryotic elongation factor 2 (EF-2), thus inhibiting myocyte protein synthesis. It may also be idiopathic. Young males are primarily affected.

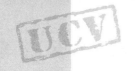

CASE 23

CARDIOLOGY

ID/CC   A 64-year-old white female complains of **sudden-onset severe pain** in her left leg with **associated weakness** of the left foot. The pain intensifies when she moves her leg, and she cannot move her toes at all.

HPI   She is a **smoker** and has a history of **limited exercise tolerance** due to **pain in her lower extremities** (INTERMITTENT CLAUDICATION).

PE   VS: normal. PE: lipid deposition in skin (XANTHELASMAS); popliteal, dorsalis pedis, and posterior tibial **pulses lost** on left side; femoral pulses easily palpable; left leg **cold and mottled; anesthesia** over lower left leg.

Labs   CBC: leukocytosis.

Imaging   US, Doppler: obstruction of left femoral artery at origin. Angio: confirmatory; assess runoff and collaterals prior to surgery.

Treatment   Thrombolysis; consider embolectomy.

Discussion   Arterial embolism may have various causes, such as **atrial fibrillation, myocardial infarction, prosthetic heart valves,** endocarditis, cancer, dilated cardiomyopathy, **paradoxical embolism** from the venous system, or a dislodged mural thrombus from an **abdominal aortic aneurysm** or an atheromatous plaque. The earlier the intervention, the higher the likelihood that the limb may be salvaged. Clinically characterized by the **five P's: pain, pallor, paralysis, paresthesia, and pulselessness.**

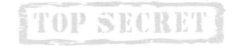

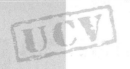

CASE 24

ID/CC   A 25-year-old male is brought to the ER after having sustained a stab wound on his left thigh following a drunken brawl.

HPI   A tourniquet was tied above the site, which the attendants said was **spurting blood like "a tap run open."**

PE   VS: **hypotension**; weak, fast pulse. PE: anxious and confused; **cool skin with reduced capillary filling**; very **low central venous pressure**; releasing tourniquet confirmed femoral artery puncture.

Labs   CBC: mildly decreased hematocrit. BUN and creatinine normal. Lytes: normal.

Imaging   Arteriogram shows abrupt termination of dye propagation in the common femoral artery.

Treatment   Arrest of femoral artery hemorrhage with vascular repair; intensive IV fluid therapy using normal saline and cross-matched blood transfusions; supplemental oxygen; close monitoring of pulse rate, blood pressure, urine output, and central venous pressure.

Discussion   The clinical conditions that cause hypovolemic shock include **acute and subacute hemorrhage and dehydration**; fluid loss into an extravascular compartment can significantly reduce intravascular volume and result in nonhemorrhagic hypovolemic shock. Acute pancreatitis, loss of the enteral integument (from conditions such as burns and surgical wounds), or occlusive or dynamic ileus can all induce oligemic hypotension as a result of extravasation of fluids into the extracellular compartment. Other forms of water and solute loss, such as diarrhea, hyperglycemia (leading to glucosuria), diabetes insipidus, salt-wasting nephritis, protracted vomiting, adrenocortical failure, acute peritonitis, and overzealous use of diuretics, can also lead to decreased intravascular volume and hypovolemic shock. Patients with prolonged tissue hypoperfusion may progress to metabolic acidosis.

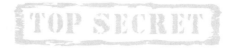

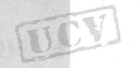

CASE 25

ID/CC
A 29-year-old-male is referred to a cardiology clinic for evaluation for a permanent pacemaker.

HPI
The patient is asymptomatic and denies dizziness, syncope, chest pain, or shortness of breath. He was incidentally noted to have **sinus bradycardia**. He is a **marathon runner** and works as a ranger in a national park, often at elevations above 8,000 feet.

PE
VS: no fever, **mild hypotension (BP 90/50) without orthostasis; bradycardia (HR 40)**. PE: thin and athletic-looking; normal JVP; S1 and S2 normally auscultated without any murmurs, gallops, and/or rubs; no lower extremity edema.

Labs
CBC/Lytes: normal. ECG: marked **sinus bradycardia** with a ventricular rate of **40 beats/minute**.

Imaging
XR, chest: normal.

Treatment
In emergent situations, treat **symptomatic sinus bradycardia** with IV access, supplemental oxygen, and cardiac monitoring. IV atropine may be used in symptomatic patients. Correct all underlying electrolyte and acid-base disorders or hypoxia. Address cause of bradycardia. This patient has a **physiologic sinus bradycardia**, and thus no treatment is indicated.

Discussion
Sinus bradycardia is defined as a sinus rhythm with a resting heart rate of less than 60 beats/minute. Physiologic causes of sinus bradycardia include **increased vagal tone** seen in athletes and incidental findings in young or sleeping patients. Pathologic causes include **inferior wall myocardial infarction, toxic or environmental exposure (dimethyl sulfoxide, toluene), electrolyte disorders, infection, sleep apnea, drug effects (digitalis glycosides, beta-blockers, amiodarone, calcium channel blockers), hypoglycemia, hypothyroidism, and increased intracranial pressure**. The most common cause of symptomatic sinus bradycardia is **sick sinus syndrome**.

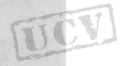

CASE 26

ID/CC   A 50-year-old male presents with complaints of **palpitations** and **chest pain**.

HPI   The pain increases with physical activity and is relieved by rest. He has **multiple sexual partners**.

PE   VS: high-volume, **collapsing pulse** (WATER-HAMMER PULSE); **wide pulse pressure**. PE: pistol shots heard over brachial artery; to-and-fro murmur heard over femoral artery (DUROZIEZ'S MURMUR); cardiomegaly; loud aortic component of S2; grade III **early diastolic murmur** heard radiating down right sternal edge (murmur of aortic incompetence); mid-diastolic murmur heard at apex (AUSTIN FLINT MURMUR).

Labs   ECG: **left ventricular hypertrophy** with strain pattern. **VDRL and FTA-ABS positive**.

Imaging   CXR: "**tree bark**" **calcification** of ascending aorta and arch of aorta; **mediastinal widening and cardiomegaly**. Echo: **aortic incompetence**; left ventricular hypertrophy and dilatation.

Gross Pathology   Gross cardiac hypertrophy (cor bovinum); **aortic aneurysm** involving the **arch** and the **ascending aorta** and extending into the aortic valve, rendering it incompetent.

Micro Pathology   **Obliterative endarteritis** of vasa vasorum; degeneration and fibrosis of outer two-thirds of aortic media; compensatory irregular fibrous thickening of aortic intima.

Treatment   Penicillin; surgical excision and repair.

Discussion   Aortitis occurs in the **tertiary stage of syphilis**, often arising many decades after the primary infection. Weakening of the aortic wall causes dilatation of the aortic root as well as aortic incompetence and aneurysms. Intimal fibrosis causes narrowing of the openings of the coronary arteries (ostial stenosis), resulting in myocardial ischemia.

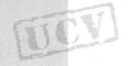

CASE 27

CARDIOLOGY

ID/CC   A 35-year-old man complains of severe, **cramping pains in his calves that prevent him from walking** (INTERMITTENT CLAUDICATION).

HPI   The patient states that the pain comes mainly after playing basketball. More recently it has appeared, accompanied by numbness, following mild exertion and **at rest** (due to progression of disease). He admits to **smoking** up to three packs of cigarettes per day.

PE   Painful, cordlike indurations of veins (sequelae of **migratory superficial thrombophlebitis**); **pallor**; cyanosis; coldness; diminished peripheral artery pulsations; **Raynaud's phenomenon**; delayed return of hand color following release of temporarily occluded radial artery while exercising hand.

Imaging   Angio, peripheral: **multiple occluded segments** of small and medium-sized arteries in lower leg.

Gross Pathology   Arterial segmental thrombosis; **no atherosclerosis**; secondary **gangrene** of leg if severe.

Micro Pathology   Segmental vasculitis with round cell infiltration in **all layers** of arterial wall; inflammation; thrombosis; microabscess formation.

Treatment   **Cessation of smoking** critical; avoidance of exposure to cold and other vasoconstriction-inducing agents; sympathectomy; amputation. Surgical revascularization is usually not possible owing to diffuse and segmental involvement and to the distal nature of the disease.

Discussion   Thromboangiitis obliterans tends to affect medium-size and small arteries of the distal extremities. If smoking is not discontinued, multiple finger and toe amputations may be necessary.

Buerger's disease

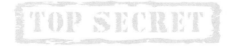

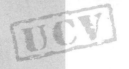

CASE 28

ID/CC
A 50-year-old female who was admitted to the hospital for treatment of staphylococcal endocarditis complains of **severe pain at the site of antibiotic infusion**.

HPI
She was receiving **cloxacillin** (has propensity to cause thrombophlebitis) in addition to penicillin and gentamycin.

PE
Markedly **tender, cordlike inflamed area** found at site of infusion.

Gross Pathology
Intraluminal venous thrombus adherent to the vessel wall.

Micro Pathology
Acute inflammatory cells with endothelial wall damage and intraluminal thrombosis.

Treatment
Change infusion site frequently; NSAIDs and local heat; support and bed rest.

Discussion
Superficial thrombophlebitis most commonly occurs in **varicose veins** or in **veins cannulated for an infusion**. Spontaneous thrombophlebitis may occur in conditions such as pregnancy, polycythemia, polyarteritis nodosa, and Buerger's disease (thromboangiitis obliterans) and as a sign of visceral cancer (thrombophlebitis migrans—Trousseau's sign).

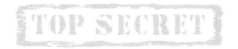

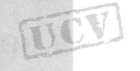

CASE 29

ID/CC
A 15-year-old boy is referred to a cardiologist by a primary care physician for an evaluation of **recurrent dizzy spells**.

HPI
During his episodes he feels **intense anxiety with palpitations and breathlessness**. He has no history of chest pain or syncope and is normal in between episodes of dizziness.

PE
General and systemic physical exam normal; cardiac exam normal; otologic causes ruled out.

Labs
ECG: **short PR interval, wide QRS complex, and a slurred upstroke** ("DELTA WAVE") of QRS complex; R wave in V1 positive. Electrophysiologic studies confirm **presence of a bypass tract** and its potential for development of life-threatening arrhythmia.

Treatment
Catheter radiofrequency ablation of the accessory tract is the treatment of choice. Since digitalis reduces the refractory period of the accessory tract, it should be avoided.

Discussion
Wolff–Parkinson–White (WPW) syndrome is a term that is applied to patients with both preexcitation on ECG and paroxysmal tachycardia; in this case, the spells of dizziness could have been either paroxysmal supraventricular tachycardia or atrial fibrillation. In WPW syndrome, an accessory pathway (Kent's bundle) exists between the atria and ventricles. An atrial premature contraction or a ventricular premature contraction generally initiates the reentrant tachycardia, with the accessory tract usually conducting in a retrograde manner; the danger of atrial fibrillation lies in the fact that the accessory pathway may be capable of conducting very fast atrial rates, leading to a fast ventricular response that may degenerate into ventricular arrhythmias.

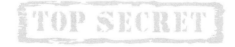

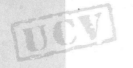

CASE 30

ID/CC   A 60-year-old white male **farmer** presents with skin lesions on his **forehead, above his upper lip, and on the dorsum of his hands.**

HPI   He does not smoke, drink alcohol, or chew tobacco.

PE   Round or irregularly shaped lesions; tan plaques with adherent **scaly or rough surface** on forehead, skin over upper lip, forearms, and dorsum of hands; lesions range in size from several millimeters to 1 cm or more.

Micro Pathology   Epidermis thickened with basal cell hyperplasia; atypical cells tend to invade most superficial portion of the dermis, which shows thickening and fibrosis (ELASTOSIS).

Treatment   Liquid-nitrogen cryotherapy; topical treatment with fluorouracil; surgical excision; electrodesiccation; minimize sun exposure.

Discussion   Also known as **senile or solar keratosis**, **actinic keratosis** is the most common **precancerous dermatosis** and may progress to **squamous cell carcinoma**. It occurs most commonly in **fair-skinned** individuals and in older persons. Signs that actinic keratosis has become malignant are elevation, ulceration or inflammation, and recent enlargement (> 1 cm). Immunosuppressed patients are at high risk of developing actinic keratosis with **prolonged sun exposure**. Look for **multiple lesions** and for newly developed lesions; **biopsy all suspicious lesions**.

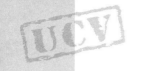

ID/CC   A 12-year-old male presents with severe **itching** and burning at the back of both knees.

HPI   He has had similar episodes since the age of 7. His **mother** suffers from **asthma** and his **father** had a **similar skin ailment**.

PE   VS: no fever. PE: perioral pallor, increased palmar markings, and **extra fold of skin below the lower eyelid** (DENNIE'S LINE); **erythematous, vesicular, weeping, rough patchy skin rash** in both popliteal fossae with thickening, crusting, and scaling on the peripheries.

Labs   CBC: **eosinophilia. High serum IgE levels.**

Micro Pathology   Skin biopsy reveals lymphocytic infiltrate with edematous intercellular spaces in the epidermis and prominent intercellular bridges; splayed keratinocytes located primarily in the stratum spinosum.

Treatment   Avoidance of skin irritants; low- or midpotency **topical glucocorticoids**; antihistamines; systemic antibiotics (for secondary infection). Severe exacerbations unresponsive to topical steroids may need systemic steroids or immunosuppressive therapy.

Discussion   Clinical criteria for the diagnosis of atopic dermatitis include recurrent episodes of pruritus lasting more than 6 weeks with a personal or family history of atopy and skin lesions typical of eczematous dermatitis.

DERMATOLOGY

TOP SECRET

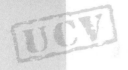
ID/CC A 68-year-old **red-haired white** male presents with a 3-month history of a progressively **raised, bleeding, ulcerated lesion** over his upper lip that has not responded to various ointments.

HPI He is a **farmer** and has always **worked outdoors**; he occasionally smokes but does not drink.

PE Large, **ill-defined, telangiectatic and ulcerated nodule** ("PEARLY PAPULE") with heaped-up borders located over right upper lip; no regional lymphadenopathy.

Gross Pathology Generally local but sometimes extensive destruction.

Micro Pathology Biopsy shows basophilic cells with scant cytoplasm as well as palisading basal cells with atypia and increased mitotic index.

Treatment Surgical excision with biopsy; cryosurgery; electrodesiccation.

Discussion Basal cell carcinoma typically occurs in **light-skinned people**. The **most common skin cancer**, it is seen mainly on **sun-exposed areas** (e.g., face, nose) and is very **slow-growing**. **Metastatic disease is rare** (< 0.17%); **chronic, prolonged exposure to sun** is the most important risk factor. Other risk factors include **male gender**, **advanced age**, **fair complexion**, and **outdoor occupations**. An increased incidence is seen in people with **defective DNA repair mechanisms** (e.g., **xeroderma pigmentosum**) and **immunosuppression**.

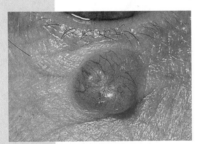

Figure 032A Pearly papule with superficial telangiectasias and a rolled border.

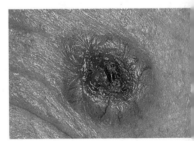

Figure 032B Pearly papule with rolled borders and central ulceration.

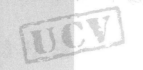

DERMATOLOGY

ID/CC
An 8-year-old boy presents with **intense pruritus and fluid-filled blisters** over his arms and legs.

HPI
He recently went on a camping trip with his classmates, during which he played the whole day in the bushes around the camping site.

PE
Typical **linear streaked vesicles over both arms and legs**; weepy and encrusted areas; numerous scratch marks over skin.

Labs
Gram stain and culture to rule out secondary infection; KOH preparation negative.

Gross Pathology
Skin erythema and edema, with linear streaked vesicles.

Micro Pathology
Superficial perivascular **lymphocytic infiltration** around the blood vessels associated with edema of the dermal papillae and mast cell degranulation.

Treatment
Systemic and oral steroids.

Discussion
While at the campground the boy probably encountered poison ivy, a plant that produces low-molecular-weight oils (URUSHIOLS) that induce contact hypersensitivity, which is a **cell-mediated, type IV hypersensitivity reaction**. The antigen is presented by the Langerhans cells to the helper lymphocytes. Both cell types travel to regional lymph nodes, where the antigen presentation is increased. Upon antigen challenge, the sensitized T-cells infiltrate the dermis and begin the immune response.

TOP SECRET

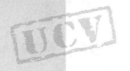

ID/CC A 35-year-old **man** presents with an **intensely pruritic rash** on his **elbows, knees, and back.**

HPI He has **celiac sprue** and observes prescribed dietary precautions (gluten restriction).

PE PE: **bilaterally symmetrical** polymorphic skin lesions in the form of **small, tense vesicles on erythematous skin** (often in herpetiform groups); bullae and groups of papules over scapular and sacral areas, knees and elbows, and other **extensor surfaces.**

Labs HLA-B8/DR-w3 haplotype (particularly prone).

Gross Pathology Polymorphous erythematous lesions, including **papules, small vesicles,** and **larger bullae.**

Micro Pathology Skin biopsy reveals characteristic **subepidermal blisters,** necrosis, and dermal papillary microabscesses; direct immunofluorescence studies reveal **granular deposits of IgA at tips of dermal papillae.**

Treatment **Dapsone therapy** after confirming adequate glucose-6-phosphate dehydrogenase (G6PD) levels (dapsone produces hemolysis in G6PD-deficient individuals).

Discussion Dermatitis herpetiformis is a vesicular and extremely pruritic skin disease associated with gluten sensitivity enteropathy and IgA immune complexes deposited in dermal papillae; individuals with HLA-B8/DR-w3 haplotype are predisposed to developing the disease. **Males** are often more commonly affected, and peak incidence is in the third and fourth decades. Patients on long-term dapsone therapy should be monitored for hemolysis and methemoglobinemia.

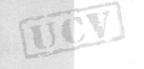
ID/CC A **16-year-old female** complains of **multiple nevi** on her skin.

HPI She is concerned because an **aunt** who had a **similar illness** developed **malignant melanoma** and died of metastatic complications.

PE Multiple nevi measuring 6 to 15 mm noted; nevi are variegated shades of pink, tan, and brown and seen on back, chest, buttocks, scalp, and breasts; **borders are irregular** and **poorly defined** but lack the scalloping of malignant melanoma; no regional lymphadenopathy noted.

Micro Pathology Skin biopsy reveals melanocytes with **cytologic and architectural atypia**, enlarged and fused epidermal nevus cell nests, **lentiginous hyperplasia**, and **pigment incontinence**.

Treatment Sun protection; regular skin exam to detect the development of malignant melanoma and for narrow-margin excisional biopsy of suspicious lesions. Family members should be regularly monitored.

Discussion Dysplastic nevi are found in individuals with an autosomal-dominant predisposition to develop acquired nevi; these **may develop into malignant melanoma**.

DERMATOLOGY

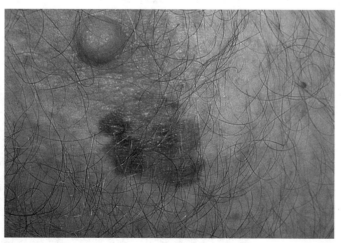

Figure 035 Asymmetric macule with irregular borders, variable color changes, and larger than 6 mm.

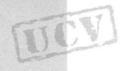

ID/CC   A 24-year-old female presents with a sudden-onset **skin rash** on both **forearms**.

HPI   She suffers from **herpes labialis** and had a recent recurrence. Currently she is not taking any medications.

PE   VS: normal. PE: **papulovesicular, erythematous skin lesions on both forearms**, occurring in **concentric rings with a clear center** (TARGET LESIONS); mucous membranes spared (vs. Stevens–Johnson syndrome).

Micro Pathology   Skin biopsy reveals dermal edema and lymphocytic infiltrates intimately associated with degenerating keratinocytes along the dermal-epidermal junction; target lesions reveal a central necrosed area with a rim of perivenular inflammation.

Treatment   **Treat underlying cause**, supportive therapy; **steroids** in severe cases.

Discussion   Erythema multiforme is a hypersensitivity response to certain **drugs** (commonly **sulfonamides, NSAIDs, penicillin, phenytoin**) and **infections** (*Mycoplasma*, HSV). It is clinically divided into major and minor types. The minor type involves limited cutaneous surfaces, while the major type (STEVENS–JOHNSON SYNDROME) is characterized by toxic features and involvement of mucosal surfaces.

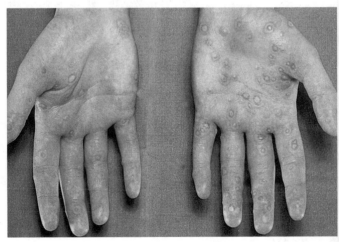

Figure 036 Multiple erythematous targetoid lesions on the palms.

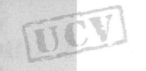

ID/CC A 24-year-old male presents with acute-onset, **painful swelling** in his **left axillae.**

HPI He also reports fever and a history of poorly controlled juvenile-onset diabetes mellitus.

PE VS: fever (39°C); tachycardia (HR 110). PE: multiple, mobile, **extremely tender, erythematous and fluctuant** axillary swellings; aspiration of swellings yields frank pus.

Labs CBC: **leukocytosis**. Gram stain of pus reveals gram-positive cocci in clusters; culture grows coagulase-positive *Staphylococcus aureus*.

Treatment **Incision and drainage**; systemic antibiotics (empiric penicillinase-resistant β-lactams; then according to reported culture sensitivities).

Discussion A boil (FURUNCLE) is a deep-seated infection of the hair follicle and adjacent subcutaneous tissue, most commonly occurring in moist hair bearing parts of the body. **Diabetes, HIV, and IV drug abuse** are predisposing conditions. Recurrent cutaneous infections with *S. aureus* may occur due to a chronic carrier state (most commonly in the anterior nares).

DERMATOLOGY

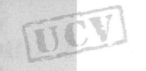

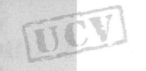

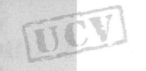TOP SECRET

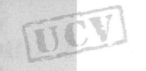37

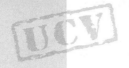

ID/CC	A 23-year-old **HIV-positive** man presents with **nonpruritic reddish-brown lesions**.
HPI	He has had a continuous low-grade fever, significant weight loss over the past 6 months, and painless lumps in the cervical, axillary, and inguinal areas.
PE	VS: fever. PE: emaciation; pallor; generalized lymphadenopathy; no hepatosplenomegaly or sternal tenderness; **reddish-purple plaques and nodules** over trunk and lower extremities; similar lesions noted in oral mucosa.
Labs	ELISA/Western blot positive for HIV. CBC/PBS: **lymphocytopenia with depressed CD4+ cell count** (< 100).
Gross Pathology	Reddish-purple, **raised plaques** and **firm nodules** with no suppuration.
Micro Pathology	Skin biopsy of nodular lesion shows malignant spindle cells with slitlike spaces containing RBCs, inflammatory cells, and hemosiderin-laden macrophages.
Treatment	Radiation; chemotherapy with etoposide or doxorubicin, bleomycin, α-interferon, and vinblastine. If iatrogenic, stop immunosuppressive medication.
Discussion	Kaposi's sarcoma is the **most common cancer associated with AIDS** (epidemic type). The non-AIDS type affects Ashkenazi Jews (chronic or classic type) and Africans (lymphadenopathic or endemic type), but the disease is not as aggressive. **Human herpesvirus 8** is associated with all types; **disordered cytokine regulation** also plays a role. Other than the skin, lesions are most commonly found in the **lymph nodes, GI tract, and lung**. In contrast to lymphoma, lymphadenopathy presents early and is not significant.

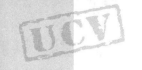

CASE 39

ID/CC
A 4-year-old Japanese male presents with **fever** and an **extensive skin rash**.

HPI
A primary care physician had previously found the patient to have cervical adenitis; antibiotics were administered but achieved no response.

PE
VS: fever. PE: **conjunctival congestion**; dry, red lips; **erythematous palms and soles**; indurative edema of peripheral extremities; **desquamation of fingertips**; various rashes of trunk; **cervical lymphadenopathy > 1.5 cm**.

Labs
Throat swab and culture sterile. CBC: routine blood counts normal; further differential blood counts reveal increased B-cell activation and T-helper-cell lymphocytopenia. Paul-Bunnell test for infectious mononucleosis negative; serologic tests rule out cytomegalovirus infection and toxoplasmosis.

Imaging
Angio: presence of **coronary artery aneurysms**.

Gross Pathology
Aneurysmal dilatation of the coronary arteries.

Micro Pathology
Coronary arteritis is usually demonstrated at autopsy together with aneurysm formation and thrombosis.

Treatment
Aspirin and IV gamma globulin are effective in preventing coronary complications if initiated early.

Discussion
Kawasaki's syndrome is usually self-limited, but in a few instances fatal coronary thrombosis has occurred during the acute stage of the disease or many months after apparently complete recovery. Case fatality rates have been about 1% to 2%.

DERMATOLOGY

TOP SECRET

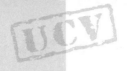

ID/CC	A 30-year-old **woman** is seen with an **itchy rash** over her **wrists, fore-arms,** and **trunk**.
HPI	She complains that fresh **lesions occur along scratch marks and areas of trauma** (KOEBNER'S PHENOMENON).
PE	VS: no fever. PE: polygonal, **purple, flat-topped papules and plaques; tiny white dots and lines over papules** (WICKHAM'S STRIAE); white netlike pattern of **lesions over oral mucosa**.
Gross Pathology	Flat-topped, **violaceous papules** and plaques **without scales**.
Micro Pathology	Dense, **bandlike (lichenoid) lymphocytic infiltrate** (predominantly T cells) along the dermal-epidermal junction; **sawtooth pattern of rete ridges**; destruction of basal cells.
Treatment	**Steroids,** topical (potent fluorinated) or systemic; psoralens with UVA therapy in refractory cases.
Discussion	Lichen planus is a **self-limited inflammatory skin** disease, but in some cases it may be present for several years. Females are affected more frequently than males. Postinflammatory hyperpigmentation may be evident after the lesions subside. Medications such as tetracycline, penicillamine, and hydrochlorothiazide can cause lichen planus–like skin reactions.

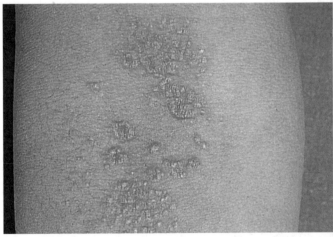

Figure 040 Persistently pruritic purplish, plane topped, polygonal papules with superficial white scale.

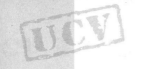
ID/CC A 50-year-old **white** male presents with an itchy, **rapidly enlarging, pigmented lesion** on the sole of his left foot.

HPI He states that the spot has **recently changed color** dramatically; once lightly pigmented, it is now a deep purple hue.

PE **Irregular, asymmetric, deeply pigmented lesion with various shades** of red and blue; diameter **> 6 mm**; left-sided nontender **inguinal lymphadenopathy**.

Gross Pathology Slightly raised; deeply pigmented with uneven hues and irregular border.

Micro Pathology Excisional biopsy shows tumor-free borders along with large, atypical, variably pigmented cells with irregular nuclei and eosinophilic nucleoli in epidermis and papillary dermis; dermal invasion noted in some places; metastases shown on lymph node biopsy.

Treatment Excision with wide margin, regional lymph node dissection, chemotherapy, immunotherapy.

Discussion Of all skin cancers, melanoma is responsible for the largest number of deaths. An increased incidence is seen in **fair-skinned** people and in those with **dysplastic nevi, immunosuppression,** and **excessive sun exposure**. Melanomas undergo a **radial (superficial) growth** phase followed by an **invasive, vertical growth** phase. **Bleeding, ulceration, and pain are late manifestations.** The **chance of metastasis increases with depth of invasion** (measured using Clark levels I–V). Metastatic melanomas are **incurable** and signify the **need for early detection** and prevention (e.g., **sunblock, clothing**).

DERMATOLOGY

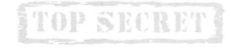

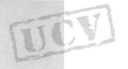

ID/CC   A 60-year-old male presents with multiple lumps and a **chronic**, pruritic, erythematous **rash** that has spread and now **involves almost his entire body**.

HPI   He has seen many doctors, but the rash **has not responded to** a variety of medications, including **topical and systemic steroids**.

PE   Erythematous, circinate rash in **plaques** with **exfoliation** (SCALING); some **nodules** seen on face, trunk, lower abdomen, and buttocks; no regional lymphadenopathy or hepatosplenomegaly.

Labs   CBC/PBS: lymphocytosis. Atypical. **PAS-positive, large, CD4-antigen-positive** (helper T-cell) **lymphocytes with characteristic multiconvoluted, "cerebriform" nuclei** (SÉZARY–LUTZNER CELLS).

Imaging   CXR: no mediastinal lymphadenopathy.

Gross Pathology   Reddish-brown, **kidney-shaped plaques** (vs. Hodgkin's lymphoma); hence name "**red man's disease**"; exfoliation, nodule formation, and sometimes ulceration.

Micro Pathology   Dermal infiltration with exocytosis of atypical mononuclear cells within epidermis found singly or within punched-out **epidermal microabscesses** (PAUTRIER'S ABSCESSES).

Treatment   Topical treatment employing PUVA; total skin electron-beam therapy; prednisone and topical chemotherapy; for advanced disease, systemic treatment with interferon, retinoids, photopheresis, and systemic chemotherapy with single agents.

Discussion   Mycosis fungoides is a malignant cutaneous helper T-cell lymphoma; disseminated disease with exfoliative dermatitis and generalized lymphadenopathy is termed Sézary syndrome.

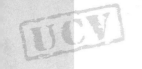

CASE 43

ID/CC A 25-year-old male is admitted to the hospital for an evaluation of **recurrent epistaxis**.

HPI The patient's mother died of a **massive pulmonary hemorrhage due to an arteriovenous malformation**.

PE **Small telangiectatic lesions** seen on lips, oral and nasal mucosa, tongue, and tips of fingers and toes; anemia noted; no pulmonary bruit heard (to detect an AV malformation).

Labs CBC: normocytic, normochromic anemia (due to occult gastrointestinal blood loss). Guaiac positive.

Imaging MR: AV malformations in liver and spleen.

Micro Pathology Irregularly dilated capillaries and venules.

Treatment **Nasal packing, cautery,** and **estrogens** may be tried to control recurrent epistaxis; significant visceral AV malformations may require embolization.

Discussion Hereditary hemorrhagic telangiectasia, or Osler-Weber-Rendu syndrome, is inherited as an **autosomal-dominant trait**. Telangiectasias may first be seen during adolescence and then increase in incidence with age, peaking between the ages of 45 and 60 years. AV fistulas may present with hemoptysis, indicating high morbidity.

DERMATOLOGY

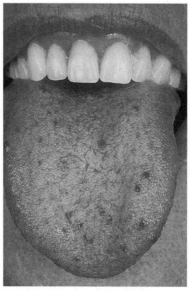

Figure 043 Multiple telangiectasias on the tongue.

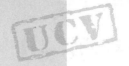
ID/CC A 45-year-old woman visits her dermatologist complaining of painful, blistering skin lesions over her back, chest, and arms that break down and leave denuded skin areas.

HPI Over the past few years she has had **large recurrent aphthous ulcers in the mouth**. She was not taking any drugs before her symptoms developed.

PE **Large aphthous ulcers** seen over oral and vaginal mucosa; **vesiculobullous skin lesions** seen in **various stages**; vertical pressure over bullae leads to **lateral extension** ("BULLA SPREAD SIGN"); skin over bullae **peels like that of a "hot tomato"** (NIKOLSKY'S SIGN).

Labs Indirect immunofluorescence test to detect antibodies in serum shows presence of IgG antibodies.

Gross Pathology Fresh vesicle is selected for biopsy.

Micro Pathology Lesions show **loss of cohesion of epidermal cells** (ACANTHOLYSIS) that produces clefts directly above basal cell layer; Tzanck smear of material from floor of a bulla reveals acantholytic cells that are round with large hyperchromatic nuclei and homogeneous cytoplasm; **direct immunofluorescence** reveals **characteristic IgG intercellular staining and deposits**.

Treatment Steroids are mainstay of therapy; cytotoxic drugs (cyclophosphamide).

Discussion **Pemphigus vulgaris**, an intraepidermal blistering disease of the skin and mucous membranes, usually appears in individuals in the third to fifth decade of life. The blisters result from loss of adhesion between epidermal cells caused by the production of autoantibodies that are directed against keratinocyte cell surface proteins; loss of cell-cell contact between desmosomes (which are sites of attachment for epidermal cells) has been demonstrated by electron microscopy. Untreated pemphigus vulgaris is often fatal.

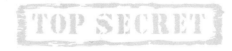

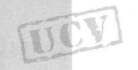

CASE 45

DERMATOLOGY

ID/CC   A 17-year-old girl presents with a **scaly rash** on her **trunk**.

HPI   Three weeks ago, she noticed a small scaly rash on her neck that progressed in about a week to involve the trunk and upper extremities. Aside from the rash, she is asymptomatic. She is sexually active.

PE   VS: normal. PE: crop of **oval, erythematous, scaly maculopapular lesions** on trunk, neck, and proximal extremities in a "**Christmas tree**" **distribution**.

Labs   RPR/VDRL non-reactive; ELISA for HIV negative.

Gross Pathology   Biopsy specimen shows **superficial perivascular dermatitis**.

Treatment   Treat with **moisturizers** and **antipruritic lotions**; **topical steroids** or **oral antihistamines** rarely required; **ultraviolet B light** used to relieve pruritus in resistant cases; provide reassurance, since disease is **benign and self-limited**, and **recurrence** is **uncommon**.

Discussion   **Pityriasis rosea** is a common skin rash with the highest incidence in young adults and teenagers. The disease is twice as common in women as in men. In most cases, the initial lesion is a 1- to 10-cm, oval maculopapular lesion, called a "**herald patch**," that is commonly found on the trunk or neck. Pityriasis rosea is a clinical diagnosis; it is important to differentiate the disease from **secondary syphilis**, **tinea versicolor**, **psoriasis**, and **drug reactions**.

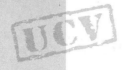

CASE 46

ID/CC A 40-year-old male comes to a dermatology outpatient clinic with an extensive, mildly pruritic, and chronic skin rash.

HPI It improves during the summer and markedly worsens in cold weather. The patient was previously diagnosed by an orthopedic surgeon with **distal interphalangeal joint arthropathy.**

PE Multiple **salmon-colored plaques** with **overlying silvery scales** seen over back and extensor aspects of upper and lower limbs; on removing scale, **underlying pinpoint bleeding capillaries** seen (AUSPITZ SIGN); lesions seen along scratch marks (KOEBNER PHENOMENA); **pitting of nails** with occasional onycholysis seen.

Imaging XR, hands: asymmetric degenerative changes involving the distal interphalangeal joints, with **"pencil-in-cup" deformity.**

Micro Pathology Skin biopsy reveals markedly thickened stratum corneum with layered zones of parakeratosis (retention of nuclei); markedly hyperplastic epidermis with elongation of rete projections; collections of PMNs within the stratum corneum (MUNRO'S MICROABSCESSES); **marked degree of epidermal hyperplasia with little inflammatory infiltrate** (characteristic microscopic finding).

Treatment Exposure to sunlight. The following have been used either alone or in combination: occlusive dressings, tar ointment, dithranol, PUVA, topical steroids, and cytotoxic drugs such as methotrexate.

Discussion Psoriasis is a hereditary condition that is characterized by well-defined plaques covered by silvery scales. Lesions are most commonly seen in an extensor distribution, but the nails, scalp, palms, and soles may also be involved; arthritis of the distal interphalangeal joint may be seen in 20% of cases. Parenteral corticosteroids are contraindicated owing to the possibility of inducing pustular lesions.

TOP SECRET

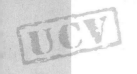

CASE 47

CC A 40-year-old female **presents** with an extremely painful **ulcer** on her left calf.

HPI The lesion appeared a month ago as a **small boil** after the patient hurt herself. It then became progressively larger until it cracked open 2 days ago. The patient reports a history of **ulcerative colitis**, which was diagnosed several years ago and managed effectively with steroid enemas and oral sulfasalazine.

PE VS: normal. PE: 10- by 10-cm deep **ulcer with violaceous border** overhanging ulcer bed; no lymphadenopathy; good distal pulses palpable (vs. arterial insufficiency ulcer); neurological exam normal.

Labs No growth demonstrated on Gram stain and culture of wound swab; **skin biopsy diagnostic**.

Micro Pathology Skin biopsy reveals hyperkeratosis; dermal perivascular round cell infiltration, and mixed infiltrate (neutrophils, lymphocytes, macrophages) extending to the subcutaneous plane.

Treatment Systemic **steroids** (oral prednisone or IV pulse methylprednisone) and **immunosuppressive** therapy (cyclosporine or tacrolimus); antibiotics for secondary infection and narcotic analgesics for pain.

Discussion Commonly associated conditions include **inflammatory bowel disease and leukemia** or **preleukemic states** (usually myelocytic leukemia or monoclonal gammopathies). Most cases occur in the fourth or fifth decades of life, with females affected slightly more often than males.

pyoderma gangrenosum

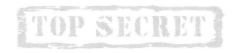

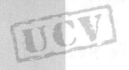

CASE 48

ID/CC A 40-year-old white male presents with a **scaly, mildly pruritic rash ove** the face and scalp.

HPI He reports that the rash is **aggravated by humidity, scratching, emo** **tional stress, and seasonal changes**. He tested **HIV positive** last yea and has since maintained a good CD4+ count without any antiretrovira therapy.

PE VS: normal. PE: interspersed thick **adherent crusts and scales** over lying areas of **greasy, yellow-red inflamed skin** involving the **scalp, fore** **head, nasolabial folds**, and **chest**.

Treatment Maintain **good hygiene; medicated shampoo**; topical **hydrocortison** **lotion** or ketoconazole cream.

Discussion A **papulosquamous skin rash** involving areas rich in sebaceous glands seborrheic dermatitis is thought to result from an **abnormal host immun** response toward a common skin commensal, *Pityrosporum ovale* Various drugs (**haloperidol, lithium, methyldopa, cimetidine**) ma worsen the condition. It is also commonly found in patients sufferin from parkinsonism and in those recovering from an acute MI.

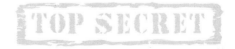

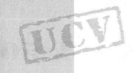

ID/CC   A 6-year-old white female is brought to the emergency room by her mother because of severe **itching, joint pain**, and a **generalized skin eruption**.

HPI   She had received an **injection of penicillin 6 days before** for streptococcal tonsillitis. Her mother denies any relevant past medical history, including allergies. Once in the hospital, the child developed fever, **edema** of the ankles and knees, hematuria, and lethargy.

PE   VS: fever. PE: generalized **urticarial skin rash**; axillary and inguinal lymphadenopathy; splenomegaly; redness and swelling of knees and ankles.

Labs   Increased ESR; decreased C3, C4 levels. UA: proteinuria; hematuria.

Gross Pathology   Generalized wheals throughout body.

Micro Pathology   Vascular lesions show fibrinoid necrosis and a neutrophilic infiltrate; **immune complex deposition in kidney and joints**.

Treatment   Antihistamines; corticosteroids; aspirin; epinephrine if severe.

Discussion   Serum sickness is a **type III hypersensitivity reaction** (immune complex disease) with a latency period between exposure to the offending agent (drugs, serum) and the appearance of signs and symptoms; it is usually self-limiting.

DERMATOLOGY

TOP SECRET

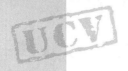

ID/CC A 19-year-old **black male** complains of **unsightly white** (depigmented) **patches** on his knees and elbows (bony prominences).

HPI He has no history of associated **pruritus** or **discomfort**. The first patch appeared over the left elbow a few months ago, and the process has been **progressive** since then.

PE PE: flat, well-demarcated areas of **depigmentation** on face (perioral or periocular), elbows, knees, and neck and in skin folds; sites of recent skin trauma are also seen to have **undergone depigmentation** (KOEBNER'S PHENOMENON); **most hairs within vitiliginous patch are white**.

Micro Pathology **Absent melanin pigment** on skin biopsy stain with ferric ferricyanide; **absence of melanocytes** on electron microscopy.

Treatment No established satisfactory treatment exists, although sunscreens protect and limit the tanning of normally pigmented skin. A promising approach is oral psoralen (a photosensitizing drug) followed by exposure to artificial long-wave ultraviolet light (UVA); potent fluorinated topical steroids may also be helpful. Generalized vitiligo may be treated by depigmentation of normal skin.

Discussion Vitiligo usually appears in otherwise-healthy persons, but several systemic disorders occur more often in patients with vitiligo, including thyroid disease (e.g., hyperthyroidism, Graves' disease, and thyroiditis) Addison's disease, pernicious anemia, alopecia areata, uveitis, and diabetes mellitus. Precipitating factors such as illness, emotional stress, or physical trauma are often associated with its onset. The disease may be inherited as an **autosomal-dominant trait** with incomplete penetrance and variable expression. Most studies, however, point to an **autoimmune** basis (circulating complement-binding anti-melanocyte antibodies have been detected).

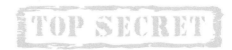

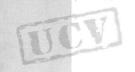

CASE 51

ID/CC A 17-year-old white male undergoing chemotherapy for disseminated Hodgkin's lymphoma complains of severe headaches, nausea, and weight loss.

HPI The patient had been on **aminoglycosides**. When questioned, he is uncertain of place and time, but despite his confusion he describes his urine as appearing reddish-orange over the past few weeks.

PE Confused but alert; underweight; no acute distress.

Labs Lytes: increased potassium. UA: hematuria; mild proteinuria; granular casts in urine; renal tubular epithelial cells in sediment; isotonic urine osmolality; **elevated urinary sodium** (> 40 mEq/L). Increased serum inorganic phosphorus; **azotemia** with BUN/creatinine ratio of 5 (within normal limits); fractional excretion of sodium > 1%.

Gross Pathology Kidneys enlarged, flabby, and pale with edema.

Micro Pathology Necrosis of tubular epithelial cells that slough into lumen, forming casts and causing blockade; hydropic degeneration of epithelium.

Treatment Discontinue offending agent; fluid and electrolyte management; renal replacement therapy with hemodialysis if indicated.

Discussion Acute tubular necrosis is defined as acute tubular damage resulting in acute renal failure; it is caused by prolonged ischemia or toxins (nephrotoxic drugs) and is usually reversible.

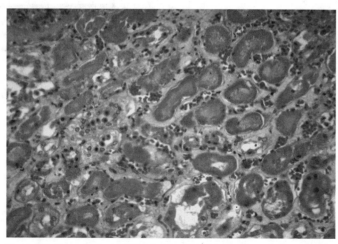

Figure 051 Necrosis of tubular epithelial cells lacking nuclei with sloughing into the tubular lumen.

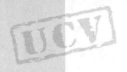
ID/CC A 47-year-old white male enters the emergency room complaining c a sudden-onset, **severe headache** that is the "**worst headache of his life.**

HPI He also describes slow-onset dull pain in his left flank and blood in hi urine. He was recently treated for **recurrent UTIs**, which were attribute to an enlarged prostate gland. His **father** died of **chronic renal failure** and his paternal **grandfather** died of **cerebral hemorrhage**.

PE VS: hypertension (BP 170/110). PE: palpable, nontender **abdomina mass** on both flanks; nuchal rigidity.

Labs UA: albuminuria; microscopic **hematuria** (no WBCs or casts). Slight increased BUN, creatinine.

Imaging Angio, neuro: ruptured **berry aneurysm**. CT/US, abdomen: **multiple kid ney and liver cysts**.

Gross Pathology Kidneys markedly enlarged and heavy with hundreds of cysts that almo: replace normal parenchyma; cysts thick-walled, ranging from a fe millimeters to several centimeters in diameter.

Micro Pathology Cystic dilatation of tubules; epithelial cell hyperplasia; cuboidal ep thelium lining cysts.

Treatment Aneurysm "clipping"; dialysis and renal transplantation.

Discussion Adult polycystic kidney disease (APKD) is an **autosomal-dominan** disease caused by a defect in chromosome 16 in which the ren; parenchyma is converted to hundreds of fluid-filled cysts, resulting i progressive renal failure in adulthood. Cysts may also involve the pai creas, liver, lungs, and spleen. It is associated with berry aneurysms the circle of Willis, hypertension, and mitral valve prolapse.

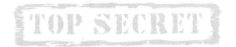

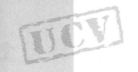

CASE 53

ID/CC A 5-year-old **female** is brought to the pediatrician because her mother noticed **blood in her urine** and **diminished vision acuity**.

HPI Her family is **Mormon**. Her mother suffers from chronic renal failure.

PE VS: BP normal. PE: appears well nourished; bilateral **sensorineural hearing loss**; bilateral **cataracts**.

Labs CBC/PBS: normochromic, normocytic **anemia**. High-tone sensorineural loss detected on audiometry; elevated serum creatinine and BUN. UA: **proteinuria**; **hematuria**; RBC casts.

Gross Pathology Small, smooth kidneys.

Micro Pathology Longitudinal thinning and splitting of glomerular basement membrane, producing characteristic laminated appearance with glomerular sclerosis; interstitial infiltrate containing fat-filled macrophages (LARGE FOAM CELLS).

Treatment ACE inhibitors; cyclosporine; renal transplantation.

Discussion Alport's syndrome can be autosomal-dominant or x-linked and is caused by a defect in the α chain of type IV collagen. It is also called hereditary chronic nephritis and is progressive in males.

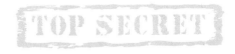

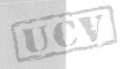

ID/CC A 45-year-old white female complains of palpitations and shortness of breath, morning swelling of the eyes, arms, and legs, and numbness of the lower legs together with weight loss and fatigue.

HPI Her past medical history is unremarkable.

PE Mild cardiomegaly; **macroglossia**; pitting **edema** in lower extremities; **ascites; cardiac arrhythmia** on auscultation.

Labs UA: proteinuria. ECG: ventricular hypertrophy and low voltage (**restrictive cardiomyopathy**). Hypoproteinemia; hyperlipidemia.

Imaging CXR: biventricular cardiac enlargement. Echo: diastolic dysfunction; increased ventricular wall thickness; increased septal thickness; granular "sparkling" appearance.

Gross Pathology Pathologic deposition of amyloid glycoprotein in several organs, primarily heart, kidney, and rectal and gingival tissue; kidneys pale, waxy, gray, and firm; spleen and liver may be enlarged; deep-brown discoloration characteristic of amyloid-infiltrated organs exposed to iodine.

Micro Pathology **Apple-green birefringence** in polarized light when stained with **Congo red**; amyloid deposition in mesangium as well as in endothelium surrounding hepatic sinusoids and in spleen; hyaline thickening of arteriolar walls, leading to narrowing of lumen and ischemia.

Treatment Supportive.

Discussion Primary amyloidosis commonly presents with nephrotic syndrome. Amyloidosis may be primary (in which the proteins are monoclonal immunoglobulin light chain) or secondary to chronic inflammatory states (especially rheumatoid arthritis and tuberculosis). The primary type is often associated with B-cell dyscrasias, especially multiple myeloma, and in these cases Bence Jones proteins are almost always present in the serum and urine.

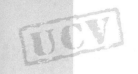

ID/CC A 56-year-old male complains of **urinary frequency** and interruption of the urinary stream over the past 6 months; he also complains of having to wake up multiple times during the night to urinate (NOCTURIA).

HPI The patient's history includes one episode of acute urinary retention one month ago that was relieved with catheterization. He denies any history of hematuria (vs. carcinoma of the bladder) or back pain (vs. metastasized prostatic carcinoma). He also admits to having a **reduced caliber of urine stream** and **terminal dribbling** as well as **urinary hesitancy**.

PE Digital rectal exam reveals **smooth enlargement of the prostate** protruding into the rectum; overlying rectal mucosa mobile; **bladder percussible up to umbilicus.**

Labs UA: 2+ bacteria; positive nitrite and leukocyte esterase. Prostate-specific antigen (PSA) levels normal; urodynamic studies demonstrate **bladder neck obstruction** with increased residual urine volume; mildly elevated serum creatinine and BUN.

Imaging US: benign-appearing enlargement of median lobe.

Gross Pathology Enlarged prostate with well-demarcated nodules up to 1 cm in diameter in **median lobe** of prostate.

Micro Pathology Both stroma and glands show **hyperplasia** on biopsy; fibromyoadenomatous hyperplasia seen in which proliferating glands are surrounded by proliferating smooth muscle cells and fibroblasts.

Treatment Finasteride alleviates symptoms by inhibiting 5α-reductase, thereby blocking androgen action on prostate; tamsulosin relieves obstruction by blocking α_1 receptors in the prostate, bladder neck, and urethra; transurethral resection of prostate (TURP).

Discussion Age-dependent changes of estrogens and androgens are believed to cause benign prostatic hypertrophy (BPH); an increasing incidence is noted starting at 40 years of age. It affects up to 75% of men by the age of 80 years.

NEPHROLOGY/UROLOGY

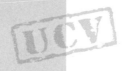

CASE 56

ID/CC	A 65-year-old **white male** complains of **painless hematuria** of several days' duration.
HPI	He is a **heavy smoker**.
PE	Lungs clear; abdomen nontender; no palpable masses; genitalia within normal limits; no lymphadenopathy.
Labs	CBC: slight normocytic, normochromic anemia. UA: **hematuria** and abundant epithelial cells.
Imaging	IVP/Cystogram: **irregular filling defects** above trigone.
Gross Pathology	Nodular, **cauliflower-like** lesion with central necrosis and minimal invasion of bladder wall.
Micro Pathology	Cytology of urine shows malignant cells. Biopsy of bladder shows grade I, stage B **transitional cell carcinoma** (TCC) arising from uroepithelium and projecting into bladder.
Treatment	Surgery (cystoprostatectomy); radiotherapy; chemotherapy.
Discussion	There is a threefold increase in risk in men, and the average age at diagnosis is 65. Risk factors for papillary carcinoma of the bladder include industrial exposure to arylamines (especially 2-naphthylamine), cigarette smoke, *Schistosoma haematobium* infection (although most *Schistosoma* infections are associated with squamous neoplasia), analgesic abuse (especially phenacetin), and long-term cyclophosphamide therapy. Complications include invasion of perivesicular tissue, ureteral invasion with urinary obstruction (leading to hydronephrosis, pyelonephritis, and renal failure), and metastases to the lung, bone, and liver. TCC appears to be associated with mutations in the p53 tumor suppressor gene and deletions in chromosomes 9p and 9q.

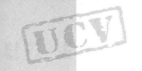

CASE 57

ID/CC   A 65-year-old male presents with **acute urinary retention**.

HPI   For the past few years, he has noted an **increased frequency** of micturition along with increased **hesitancy, urgency**, decreased force and stream of urine, and a feeling of **incomplete evacuation** of the bladder. For the past few months he has begun to experience **increasing fatigability and lassitude**.

PE   Pallor; bladder full on abdominal examination; rectal exam reveals **grade III prostate enlargement**.

Labs   CBC: normocytic anemia. Lytes: hypocalcemia; hyperphosphatemia. **Elevated BUN and creatinine**. UA: proteinuria; **no RBCs or casts seen**.

Imaging   US, kidneys: **bilateral hydroureter and hydronephrosis**.

Micro Pathology   In addition to hydronephrosis and hydroureter, interstitial kidney disease is seen on microscopic examination.

Treatment   **Transurethral resection** of the prostate (TURP) to relieve the obstruction is the basic and most useful step.

Discussion   Obstructive nephropathy results from the **impaired outflow of urine** but may also **produce chronic interstitial damage**. Obstructive nephropathy is common in childhood (from congenital abnormalities) and in individuals older than 60 years, when benign prostatic hypertrophy and prostatic and gynecologic cancers become more common.

NEPHROLOGY/UROLOGY

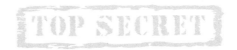

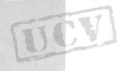

CASE 58

ID/CC   A 48-year-old white female is admitted to the hospital because of worsening **generalized edema** and weakness along with **hypertension**.

HPI   She has a long history of type I **diabetes mellitus** but no history of hematuria, recent sore throat, or skin infections.

PE   VS: hypertension (BP 160/110). PE: **generalized pitting edema**; no evidence of pleural effusion or ascites; lung bases clear on auscultation; JVP normal; neither kidney palpable; funduscopic exam reveals presence of **proliferative diabetic retinopathy**.

Labs   **Elevated** fasting **blood sugar** (234 mg/dL); elevated glycosylated hemoglobin (10%); **elevated BUN and serum creatinine; decreased serum albumin; elevated blood cholesterol**. UA: presence of sugar and **3+ protein; broad casts** and **fatty casts**; elevated quantitative protein (3.5 gm/24 hr).

Micro Pathology   **Increased mesangial matrix** on renal biopsy; **thickening of capillary basement membrane** combined with acellular eosinophilic nodules in mesangium (KIMMELSTIEL-WILSON DISEASE); hyaline arteriosclerosis of both afferent and efferent arterioles; no immune complex deposits seen.

Treatment   Blood sugar control; ACE inhibitor or angiotensin receptor blocker to help prevent progression of diabetic nephropathy; control of systemic hypertension; dietary protein and phosphate restriction; avoidance of nephrotoxic drugs; dialysis or renal transplantation.

Discussion   Diabetic glomerulosclerosis is a renal manifestation of diabetic microangiopathy and presents at least 10 years after diabetes appears (more commonly in IDDM); it is usually the prelude to end-stage diabetic renal disease.

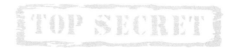

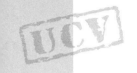

CASE 59

ID/CC	A 25-year-old white **male** complains of a chronic cough of several months' duration, accompanied by lightheadedness, fatigue, and malaise; yesterday he **coughed up blood.**
HPI	He also describes intermittent fever and headaches in addition to small volumes of **dark orange urine.** He denies alcohol use but admits to being a heavy **smoker.**
PE	Diffuse pulmonary crackles bilaterally.
Labs	Azotemia. UA: oliguria; **hematuria**; proteinuria. **Iron deficiency anemia**; blood detected in sputum. ABGs: hypoxemia. **Anti–glomerular basement membrane antibodies** in serum.
Imaging	CXR: bilateral alveolar infiltrates.
Gross Pathology	Increase in weight of lungs with areas of necrosis; **kidneys** enlarged and pale with decreased consistency.
Micro Pathology	Kidney biopsy shows proliferative, necrotizing, **crescentic glomerulonephritis** with accumulation of neutrophils and macrophages in Bowman's capsule; characteristic **linear IgG deposits in glomerular basement membrane and alveolar septa** on immunofluorescence; necrotizing hemorrhagic **alveolitis** on lung biopsy.
Treatment	Plasma exchange; corticosteroids; immunosuppressive therapy.
Discussion	Goodpasture's syndrome is hemorrhagic alveolitis with nephritis and iron deficiency anemia caused by anti-glomerular basement membrane antibodies (type II hypersensitivity reaction).

NEPHROLOGY/UROLOGY

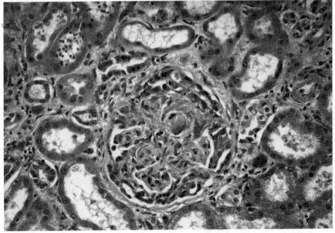

Figure 059 Epithelial crescent and cellular mesangium within the glomerulus.

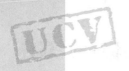
ID/CC   A 45-year-old **black** male presents with uncontrolled **hypertension** and complains of severe occipital headache and ringing in his ears.

HPI   He also reports **markedly diminished urine output over the past 24 hours.** On directed questioning, he also reports **some visual blurring.**

PE   VS: **severe hypertension.** PE: funduscopy reveals presence of **papilledema** with **hypertensive retinopathy.**

Labs   UA: proteinuria; microscopic hematuria; **red cell casts.** Elevated BUN and creatinine. CBC: microangiopathic hemolytic anemia. ECG: left-axis deviation with left ventricular hypertrophy.

Imaging   Echo: concentric left ventricular hypertrophy with reduced ejection fraction. US, abdomen: presence of **parenchymal renal disease in normal-sized kidneys** (unlike that of benign nephrosclerosis, where there are bilateral contracted kidneys).

Micro Pathology   Pathologic changes include **fibrinoid necrosis of arterioles** (NECROTIZING ARTERIOLITIS), **hyperplastic arteriolosclerosis** ("ONION SKINNING"), and necrotizing glomerulitis associated with a thrombotic microangiopathy.

Treatment   Reduction of diastolic blood pressure to at least 100 mmHg; maintain **urine output > 20 mL/hour.** Multiple medications, including labetalol, hydralazine, nitroprusside, and enalaprilat, can be used to acutely lower blood pressure.

Discussion   **Sodium nitroprusside** is the safest and most effective drug for use in hypertensive emergencies; because it does not impair myocardial blood flow, it is especially useful in underlying ischemic heart disease. However, it is metabolized to cyanide and thiocyanate; therefore, prolonged use may lead to cyanide toxicity or to thiocyanate toxicity. Blood thiocyanate levels should be determined frequently.

hypertensive renal disease

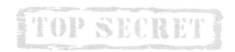

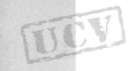

CASE 61

ID/CC A 22-year-old white male complains of recurrent episodes of "**bloody urine**" that lasted for several days **in conjunction** with a URI.

HPI He was well until the onset of symptoms.

PE Pallor; slight palpebral edema.

Labs UA: proteinuria; **red cell casts in urine**; gross hematuria. **Increased serum IgA.**

Micro Pathology Focal glomerulonephritis involving only selected glomeruli with **mesangial proliferation** and segmental necrosis with crescents; immunofluorescence typically reveals mesangial **IgA deposits** with some IgM, IgG, and C3.

Treatment Supportive; ACE inhibitors for hypertension and proteinuria; fish oil; immunosuppressive therapy in selected cases; IgA deposits commonly reappear following kidney transplantation.

Discussion IgA nephropathy is idiopathic but associated with upper respiratory or GI infections lacking a latency period (vs. poststreptococcal glomerulonephritis). Lesions are variable and may be mesangioproliferative, focal proliferative, or possibly crescentic glomerulonephritis. The glomerular pathology seen in Berger's disease is similar to that seen in Henoch–Schönlein purpura, which is seen in children. It is seen with increased frequency in patients with celiac disease and liver disease (due to defective IgA clearance). Chronic renal failure may ultimately develop.

NEPHROLOGY/UROLOGY

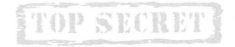

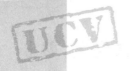
ID/CC   A **30-year-old black woman** presents with **pain** in both her knee **joints** and in the small joints of the hand together with mild fever, anorexia, weight loss, and loss of hair.

HPI   She also has a history of **recurrent oral ulcerations** and a **photosensitive skin rash**. No joint deformities are reported.

PE   VS: hypertension. PE: oral **aphthous ulcers** noted; erythematous **photosensitive skin rash**; "**butterfly rash**" over malar area of face; pallor; no abdominal or renal bruits heard.

Labs   CBC: normocytic, normochromic **anemia**. UA: microscopic hematuria with **RBC casts** in addition to proteinuria. **Elevated BUN and creatinine; antinuclear antibodies positive** in high titer; **LE cell phenomenon** positive; **anti-Sm antibody and anti-ds DNA antibody positive; VDRL positive** but FTA-ABS negative; low serum complement levels.

Micro Pathology   Renal biopsy reveals features of **diffuse proliferative glomerulonephritis**. Electron microscopy reveals **immune complex deposits** that are typically **subendothelial** and form "**wire loops**."

Treatment   Corticosteroids; cytotoxic drugs (cyclophosphamide, azathioprine, and chlorambucil); long-term hemodialysis or transplant.

Discussion   There are five patterns of lupus nephritis. Class I is normal by light, EM, and immunofluorescence microscopy. Class II presents as **mesangial lupus glomerulonephritis** and is found in about 25% of patients; it is associated with minimal hematuria or proteinuria. Class III is characterized by **focal proliferative** glomerulonephritis and is associated with recurrent hematuria and mild renal insufficiency. Class IV is described in this case and is by far the most common form. Class V presents as **membranous glomerulonephritis** and is seen in 15% of cases; it induces severe proteinuria or nephrotic syndrome.

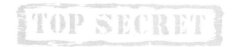

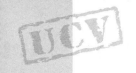

CASE 63

ID/CC An 11-year-old white girl is brought to the pediatrician because of headache, chest palpitations, and ringing in her ears together with **generalized edema**.

HPI She has no history of dyspnea, sore throat, skin infections, or fever. Careful questioning reveals that she has also had **hematuria**.

PE VS: hypertension (BP 140/100). PE: **generalized** (including periorbital) **pitting edema**; JVP normal; lung bases clear; neither kidney palpable; no evidence of pleural effusion or ascites.

Labs Elevated BUN and serum creatinine; decreased serum albumin; elevated serum triglycerides; serum **hypocomplementemia**; antinuclear antibody (ANA) negative; normal ASO titers. UA: **fatty casts and oval bodies in addition to proteins**.

Micro Pathology Diffuse glomerular involvement with thickened capillary walls and lobular mesangial proliferation on light microscopy. **Splitting of basement membrane causing railroad-track appearance** with PAS reagent or silver stain; **prominent granular immunofluorescence**; mesangial and subendothelial deposits of immune complexes.

Treatment Corticosteroids; renal transplantation.

Discussion Membranoproliferative glomerulonephritis (MPGN) is idiopathic but may be associated with inherited deficiencies of complement components and partial lipodystrophy. It is subdivided into two types: type I MPGN (both classic and alternative complement pathways activated) and type II MPGN (dense deposit disease; activation of alternate complement pathway). The majority of patients with MPGN will go on to develop **chronic renal failure**. There is a **high recurrence rate** following renal transplantation.

NEPHROLOGY/UROLOGY

TOP SECRET

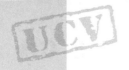

ID/CC	A 47-year-old black diabetic female complains of weight loss, progressive shortness of breath, and **swelling of the lower legs** and arms.
HPI	Her past medical history is unremarkable.
PE	Pallor; pitting edema in extremities; decreased lung sounds with crackles bilaterally in lower lung fields; **periorbital edema; ascites**.
Labs	UA: **proteinuria** (> 3.5 g/24 hr); lipiduria with oval fat bodies and fatty and waxy casts in urinary sediment. **Hypoalbuminemia** (< 3 g/dL); **hyperlipidemia** (serum cholesterol 250 mg/dL).
Gross Pathology	Kidneys enlarged, pale, and rubbery; renal vein thrombosis may be present.
Micro Pathology	Thickened **basement membrane**; subepithelial deposits of IgG and C3 along basement membrane seen in **"spike and dome"** pattern on methenamine silver stain; immune deposits in a **"lumpy-bumpy"** (discontinuous) pattern on immunofluorescence.
Treatment	Corticosteroids; cyclophosphamide; renal transplantation; ACE inhibitors reduce urinary protein loss.
Discussion	Nephrotic syndrome may be idiopathic or caused by membranous glomerulonephritis (the most common cause in adults), minimal change disease (LIPOID NEPHROSIS) (the most common in children), focal glomerulosclerosis, or membranoproliferative glomerulonephritis. Patients with nephrotic syndrome have hypercoagulability secondary to loss of antithrombin III in the urine (e.g., increased incidence of peripheral vein thrombosis).

membranous glomerulonephritis

TOP SECRET

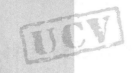

CASE 65

ID/CC   A **5-year-old** white male presents with **generalized edema** and abdominal distention, producing respiratory embarrassment.

HPI   The child had a **URI** 1 week ago.

PE   VS: BP normal. PE: generalized pitting edema; free **ascitic fluid** in peritoneal cavity; shifting dullness and fluid thrill present; normal funduscopic exam.

Labs   UA: 4+ proteinuria (> 3 g/24 h). **Hypoalbuminemia; hypercholesterolemia**; hypertriglyceridemia; decreased serum ionic calcium; normal C3 levels; normal serum creatinine and BUN.

Gross Pathology   Kidneys slightly enlarged, soft, and yellowish.

Micro Pathology   Light microscopy and immunofluorescent studies **normal on renal biopsy** (no evidence of immune complex deposition). EM reveals uniform and diffuse loss of the podocytic foot processes.

Treatment   **Corticosteroids**; salt-restricted diet; diuretics; electrolyte therapy and monitoring.

Discussion   Also called **lipoid nephrosis**, minimal change disease is the most common cause of idiopathic **nephrotic syndrome in children** and is associated with infections or vaccinations. It carries a **good prognosis**.

Figure 065 Periorbital edema, abdominal distension, and bilateral lower extremity edema (anasarca).

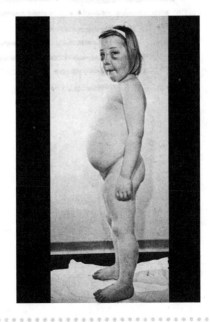

NEPHROLOGY/UROLOGY

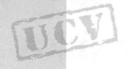
ID/CC   A 68-year-old **black** male complains of **dysuria, progressively increased** urinary frequency, and **back pain** that has lasted several months.

HPI   He reports **high animal-fat intake**.

PE   Nodular, **rock-hard, irregular area of induration** in peripheral lobe of prostate on digital rectal exam; **midline furrow** between prostatic lobes **obscured; extension to seminal vesicles** detected.

Labs   **Markedly elevated prostate-specific antigen** (PSA) and **acid phosphatase**.

Imaging   Transrectal US, prostate: **hypoechoic masses** in peripheral zone with extension to seminal vesicles. Nuc, bone scan: **hot lesions of spine, sacrum, and pelvic bones** (axial skeleton). CT/MR: prostate mass with capsular penetration and enlarged seminal vesicles.

Gross Pathology   Irregularly enlarged, firm, nodular prostate.

Micro Pathology   Core needle biopsy of prostate reveals single layer of malignant neoplastic cells arranged haphazardly in adenoplastic stroma.

Treatment   Prostatectomy with radiation; orchiectomy; leuprolide; antiandrogens such as flutamide.

Discussion   A primary malignant neoplasm of the prostate commonly arising from the peripheral zone (70%), prostate carcinoma is the **most common male cancer**. Its prognosis and treatment depend heavily on **stage**. Most cases are diagnosed in **asymptomatic** men on digital rectal exam. Prostate cancer exhibits **hematogenous dissemination**, most commonly to **bone**, forming **osteoblastic lesions**. The tumor can also invade sacral nerve roots, causing significant pain.

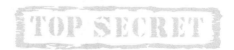

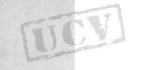

CASE 67

ID/CC	A 60-year-old white male complains of right **flank pain** and **hematuria**.
HPI	He has been a **heavy smoker** for the past 24 years; he **lost 5 pounds over the past month** and is not on a diet.
PE	VS: low-grade fever; moderate hypertension. PE: pallor; **palpable mass** in right flank.
Labs	Elevated ESR. CBC/PBS: normocytic, normochromic **anemia**. UA: gross **hematuria**.
Imaging	IVP/CT/US: mass in upper pole of right kidney. MR: no invasion of renal vein or inferior vena cava (IVC).
Gross Pathology	Yellowish areas of necrotic tissue with focal areas of hemorrhage within renal parenchyma.
Micro Pathology	Polygonal **clear cells** (containing glycogen) with evidence of cytologic atypia invading renal parenchyma.
Treatment	Right **nephrectomy**; consider renal-sparing partial nephrectomy; chemotherapy, immunotherapy, and radiation treatment may be considered for advanced or metastatic disease.
Discussion	The **most common renal tumor**, renal cell carcinoma is frequently sporadic but is seen in association **with von Hippel-Lindau syndrome** and **dialysis-related acquired polycystic kidney disease**. It frequently invades the **renal vein and IVC** and metastasizes to lungs and bone via hematogenous dissemination. It can also cause **paraneoplastic syndromes** (secondary to the production of erythropoietin, parathyroid-like hormone, ACTH, and renin).

NEPHROLOGY/UROLOGY

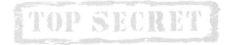

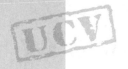

ID/CC A 63-year-old white male complains of **sudden-onset pain** in the right **flank** together with gross **hematuria**, nausea, and vomiting.

HPI He is **overweight**, has been diabetic for 15 years, is a heavy **smoker** and drinker, and has been surgically treated for **aortofemoral occlusive disease** (graft).

PE VS: no fever; mild hypertension (BP 150/100). PE: **acute distress**; pallor; sweating; severe right flank pain; **xanthelasma** in both eyelids.

Labs Normal BUN and creatinine. UA: **hematuria**. ECG: old silent anterior wall myocardial infarction. Elevated **LDH**.

Imaging CT, abdomen: **wedge-shaped, nonenhancing lesion in right kidney**. US, renal: edematous kidney with focal region of decreased color flow.

Gross Pathology Pale, yellowish-white, wedge-shaped area with hemorrhagic necrosis in renal cortex.

Micro Pathology Coagulation necrosis involving renal cortical nephrons extending into corticomedullary junction.

Treatment Remove arterial obstruction by thrombolysis; heparin anticoagulation to prevent recurrence.

Discussion Risk factors for embolic events include atherosclerosis and mural thrombi in the heart and aorta, infectious endocarditis vegetations, and atheromatous plaques in the aorta. Complications from renal artery embolism include renal failure, hypertension, acute pyelonephritis, and renal abscess.

renal infarction

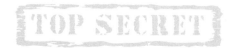

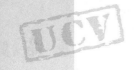

CASE 69

ID/CC   A **30-year-old** white female is found to be **hypertensive** on routine physical exam.

HPI   She claims to have **no history of hypertension** and denies any changes in lifestyle or excessive stress.

PE   VS: **hypertension** (BP 175/105). PE: loud S2; funduscopic exam normal; **abdominal bruit** present.

Labs   **Elevated plasma renin**; hypokalemia.

Imaging   Angio, renal: confirmatory; unilateral left **renal artery stenosis in a "string of pearls" pattern.**

Gross Pathology   In fibromuscular dysplasia, the renal artery lumen is decreased due to hyperplastic fibrotic wall thickening.

Micro Pathology   Muscular hyperplasia with fibrosis and segmental stenosis.

Treatment   **ACE inhibitors** (contraindicated in bilateral renal artery stenosis); calcium channel blockers; balloon angioplasty; stenting; surgical correction.

Discussion   Renovascular hypertension is secondary systemic hypertension caused by hypersecretion of renin from hypoperfused kidney(s). It is most often caused by **fibromuscular dysplasia (young Caucasian women)** or **atherosclerosis (older men)** and accounts for < 5% of all causes of hypertension.

NEPHROLOGY/UROLOGY

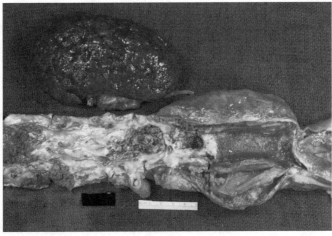

Figure 069 Shrunken kidney with a granular capsule adjacent to aorta with atherosclerosis.

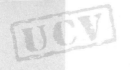

ID/CC	A 36-year-old white male presents with **progressive painless enlargement of the left testicle** of 2 months' duration.
HPI	He also complains of a sense of heaviness in his scrotum. He denies any history of pain or trauma at the site.
PE	Walnut-sized, nontender, smooth, **firm mass at upper end of left testicle; mass does not transilluminate**; epididymis and vas deferens normal on palpation; prostate and seminal vesicles normal on digital rectal exam; abdominal lymph nodes not palpable; no hepatomegaly.
Labs	Normal levels of hCG; **normal levels of serum α-fetoprotein and LDH; histologic** diagnosis based on postoperative specimen study.
Imaging	CXR: no metastasis. US, abdomen and pelvis/scrotum: solid intratesticular mass. CT, abdomen and pelvis: no metastasis.
Gross Pathology	Solid white bulging mass within testis.
Micro Pathology	Sheets of germ cells containing clear cytoplasm with lymphocytes in fibrous stroma.
Treatment	Orchiectomy followed by retroperitoneal lymph node dissection; chemotherapy with cisplatin; radiotherapy.
Discussion	Seminoma is the most common type of germ cell tumor. Dysgerminomas in ovaries are histologically similar. Tumors are extremely radiosensitive. It is associated with a good prognosis. Cryptorchidism predisposes to the development of testicular tumors.

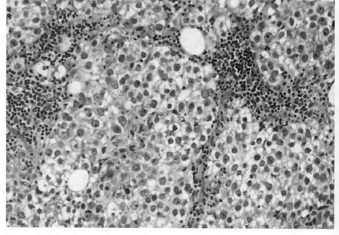

Figure 070 Solid nests of germ cells surrounded by fibrous stoma containing lymphocytes.

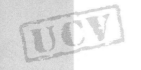

CASE 71

ID/CC A 30-year-old man complains of a small **painless nodular swelling over his right testicle** that he noticed a few months ago, coupled with **increasing growth of his breast tissue**.

HPI He also complains of mild shortness of breath on exertion (DYSPNEA), cough, and blood-streaked sputum.

PE VS: normal. PE: bilateral gynecomastia (breast tissue palpable); small, **pea-shaped swelling** involving the **right testicle**; testicular sensation lost; no transillumination; **left supraclavicular lymphadenopathy**; hepatomegaly.

Labs CBC: mild anemia. Serum β-hCG elevated.

Imaging CXR: two "cannonball" parenchymal masses (due to metastases). CT, abdomen: enlarged retroperitoneal lymph nodes and multiple hepatic metastases. US, scrotum: complex, solid right testicular mass.

Gross Pathology Small, pea-shaped hemorrhagic mass seen in right testicle.

Micro Pathology Polygonal, comparatively uniform **cytotrophoblastic cells** with clear cytoplasm growing in sheets and cords, mixed with **multinucleate syncytiotrophoblastic cells** that have **eosinophilic vacuolated cytoplasm** with readily **demonstrable hCG**; no well-developed villi seen.

Treatment **Chemotherapy** with **cisplatin, etoposide, and bleomycin** in some combination, followed by **radical inguinal orchiectomy** and **retroperitoneal lymph node dissection**; gynecomastia regresses once the source of hCG (the tumor) is removed.

Discussion Choriocarcinoma is the **most malignant of all testicular tumors**; it metastasizes relatively early via both the **lymphatics** and the **bloodstream** even when it remains very small locally. Follow up with β-hCG levels.

NEPHROLOGY/UROLOGY

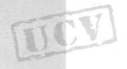

CASE 72

ID/CC	A newborn baby is evaluated for **ambiguous external genitalia**.
HPI	The baby was delivered vaginally at full term without any pre-, intra-, or postnatal complications; the mother did not take **hormones** or any other **drugs during pregnancy**.
PE	Incompletely **virilized external genitalia**; hypospadias; **bilateral inguinal swelling**.
Labs	Karyotype: **46,XY. Müllerian structures absent**; inguinal swellings proved to be **maldescended dysgenetic testes**.
Imaging	US: absence of müllerian structures and presence of dysgenic testes.
Micro Pathology	Testes characterized by **seminiferous tubule degeneration** and invasion by connective tissue arranged in whorls.
Treatment	**Gonadectomy** to protect against increased risk of testicular tumor; **hormone replacement** therapy given at puberty.
Discussion	The incidence of **gonadal tumors in dysgenetic gonads** may reach up to 30%, making orchiectomy and subsequent hormone replacement the best therapeutic option.

testicular dysgenesis

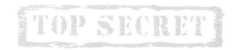

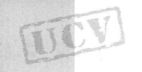
ID/CC   A 23-year-old **white** male is seen by his family physician because of **dyspnea, bilateral enlargement of the breasts** (GYNECOMASTIA), and a **painless lump in the right testis** of approximately 2 months' duration.

HPI   He denies any history of STDs, genital ulcers, drug use, or trauma.

PE   Bilateral nontender gynecomastia (due to increased hCG); left supra-clavicular lymphadenopathy; 5-cm **hard mass** palpable **on right testis**, distorted shape; normal rectal exam.

Labs   **Markedly elevated blood hCG and α-fetoprotein (AFP).**

Imaging   US/MR, testes: **solid intratesticular mass** with some foci of hemorrhage (intratesticular masses usually malignant). CT, chest, abdomen, and pelvis (for staging disease): paracaval and interaortocaval lymphadenopathy.

Micro Pathology   Cytotrophoblastic and syncytiotrophoblastic cells with hCG demonstrable within cytoplasm.

Treatment   High radical inguinal orchiectomy followed by retroperitoneal lymph node dissection and cisplatin-based combination chemotherapy in selected cases.

Discussion   Testicular cancer may be pure or mixed (mixed germ cell neoplasm) and is highly malignant with early and widespread metastasis. It is the most common neoplasm in men aged 20 to 35. Yolk sac tumors produce only AFP, whereas choriocarcinomas produce only hCG.

testicular teratoma (mixed)

NEPHROLOGY/UROLOGY

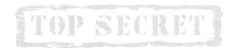

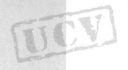

CASE 74

ID/CC   A 9-year-old black male is brought into the emergency room because of **sudden-onset** severe **pain** that he experienced in the lower abdomen and **scrotum** while playing soccer.

HPI   He has no relevant medical history. Upon admission, he became nauseated and vomited three times.

PE   Irritability; right **testicle tender, swollen**, and elevated; palpable normal epididymis anteriorly; **increased pain with elevation of mass** (PREHN'S SIGN); no hernia palpable; no transillumination of mass.

Labs   UA: mild leukocytosis.

Imaging   US, scrotum: asymmetric decreased color flow in testicle. Nuc-Tc99: **doughnut sign** (due to central testicular ischemia and circumferential collateral flow).

Gross Pathology   Testicle markedly enlarged with hemorrhagic necrosis; scrotum may be purplish; cord twisted.

Micro Pathology   Severe venous congestion; interstitial hemorrhage; hemorrhagic necrosis.

Treatment   **Immediate surgery** (detorsion and fixation of testis to scrotum) due to risk of testicle loss (less than 4 hours); contralateral orchiopexy prophylactically (high incidence of bilaterality); atrophic testicle should be removed due to possible autoimmune destruction of contralateral testis.

Discussion   Testicular torsion is a surgical emergency that needs to be differentiated from orchitis, epididymitis, and strangulated hernia. It is seen more frequently in an **undescended testicle** (CRYPTORCHIDISM); therefore, patients with cryptorchidism warrant close follow-up and perhaps corrective surgery.

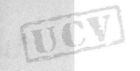

CASE 75

ID/CC
A 45-year-old man with a high-grade **non-Hodgkin's lymphoma** develops **oliguria, severe malaise,** and **fatigue** 36 hours following **chemotherapy treatment.**

PE
Carpopedal **spasm** present; neither kidney is palpable; urinary bladder is empty.

Labs
Lytes: hyperkalemia, **hyperuricemia**, and hyperphosphatemia with secondary hypocalcemia. **BUN and creatinine elevated.** UA: acidic urine with numerous **rhomboid crystals**; no casts or cells seen.

Treatment
Maintenance of good hydration, brisk alkaline diuresis, and **pretreatment with allopurinol** are keys to prevention of this syndrome; once acute renal failure has developed, fluid and electrolyte balance must be maintained and dialysis may be necessary.

Discussion
Tumor lysis syndrome is most often seen in patients with **lymphoma or leukemia** but is also seen in patients with a variety of solid tumors. The presence of a **large tumor burden, a high growth fraction, an increased pretreatment LDH level and uric acid level**, or preexisting renal insufficiency increases the likelihood that a patient will develop tumor lysis syndrome. Increased levels of uric acid, xanthine, and phosphate may result in precipitation of these substances in the kidney. Renal sludging and acute renal insufficiency or failure further aggravate the metabolic abnormality.

urate nephropathy

NEPHROLOGY/UROLOGY

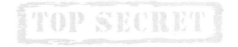

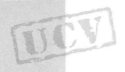

CASE 76

ID/CC   A **3-year-old** male is brought to his pediatrician for evaluation of an **abdominal mass** that his parents noticed.

HPI   The child has been well all his life.

PE   Slight pallor; weight and height within normal range; nontender, large, firm, and smooth intra-abdominal mass to right of midline; right **cryptorchidism** and **aniridia**.

Labs   UA: microscopic **hematuria**; normal urinary vanillylmandelic acid (VMA); BUN increased; serum erythropoietin elevated.

Imaging   IVP: displacement and distortion of right pelvicaliceal system. CT, abdomen: tumor arising from right kidney with areas of low density (due to necrosis); persistent ellipsoid area of enhancement (due to compressed renal parenchyma); no evidence of vascular invasion.

Gross Pathology   Whitish, solid tumor with areas of hemorrhagic necrosis distorting normal renal parenchyma compressed into narrow rim; may be involvement of perirenal fat; metastasis usually to lungs.

Micro Pathology   Glomeruloid and tubular structures enclosed within spindle cell stroma; areas of cartilage, bone, or striated muscle tissue.

Treatment   Surgical removal of kidney containing tumor; chemotherapy with actinomycin D and vincristine; radiotherapy.

Discussion   Nephroblastoma (Wilms' tumor) is a malignant tumor of embryonal origin. It is associated with deletions on chromosome 11p involving the WT-1 gene and should be differentiated from neuroblastoma and malignant lymphoma, which are other small cell tumors of childhood. Most cases are sporadic and are not associated with genetic syndromes or a positive family history. **WAGR syndrome** consists of Wilms' tumor, aniridia, genitourinary abnormalities, and mental retardation.

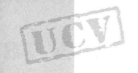

CASE 77

ID/CC   A **14-year-old male** is admitted to the hospital complaining of **pain** and **swelling** in the left **leg**.

HPI   The pain has been present for 2 months but has become progressively worse over that period. There is no history of trauma or infection.

PE   VS: **mild fever**. PE: tenderness and fusiform swelling over left femur.

Labs   Elevated ESR. Karyotype: **translocation of the long arms of chromosomes 11 and 22**.

Imaging   XR, left femur: lytic lesion in medullary zone of midshaft with cortical destruction and **"onion-skin"** appearance. CXR: no evidence of metastatic spread.

Gross Pathology   Large areas of bone lysis as tumors erode cancellous trabeculae of long bones outward to cortex.

Micro Pathology   Biopsy of bone reveals sheets of uniform, small cells resembling lymphocytes; in many places tumor cells surround a central clear area, forming a **"pseudorosette."** Cell origin of tumor is **unknown**.

Treatment   **"Melt"** tumor with radiotherapy; surgical resection; chemotherapy; regular follow-up for recurrence.

Discussion   Diaphysis of the long bones is the most common site of occurrence of Ewing's sarcoma. Five-year survival is 70% for locally resectable disease but only 30% for those with advanced metastasis.

ORTHOPEDIC

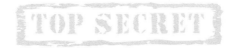

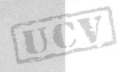

ID/CC	A 45-year-old woman visits an orthopedist because of an **inability to extend her fourth and fifth fingers**.
HPI	She has a long-standing history of **alcohol abuse** and has been to the emergency room several times for alcoholic gastritis.
PE	Mild icterus; palmar erythema; muscle wasting; malnourishment; abdomen reveals 2+ ascitic fluid (due to alcoholic liver damage); **fourth and fifth fingers of right hand reveal flexion contracture** with nodular thickening and thick bands of tissue palpable upon drawing examining finger across palm.
Gross Pathology	Infiltration of palmar fascia with fibrous tissue and subsequent contraction deformity.
Micro Pathology	Infiltration of pretendinous fascia with myofibroblasts with fibrosis of pretendinous bands.
Treatment	Surgery (release of contractures and adhesions); frequently recurs.
Discussion	Also called palmar fibromatosis, Dupuytren's contracture is of unknown etiology but is associated with alcoholism and **manual labor**. It is associated with diabetes and anticonvulsant medications.

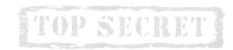

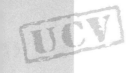

CASE 79

ID/CC

A 60-year-old woman is brought to the orthopedic clinic with complaints of **pain in the left hip and inability to bear weight** on the left leg.

HPI

Three years ago she sustained a **fracture of the neck of the femur** that was treated with internal fixation. She is an **alcoholic** and has been taking **oral steroids** for many years for a chronic skin ailment.

PE

All movements at left hip are restricted by pain; unable to bear weight on the limb.

Imaging

XR, left hip: **increase in bone density of femoral head** and collapse of articular surface; dynamic hip screw in place. MR, hip: more sensitive; decreased subchondral signal intensity and formation of reactive zones.

Treatment

Total hip replacement arthroplasty significantly reduces morbidity.

Discussion

Fracture of the neck of the femur is the most common cause of avascular necrosis of the femoral head; other risk factors include **excessive alcohol consumption, steroid therapy, radiation therapy, sickle cell anemia**, and **deep sea diving (Caisson's disease)**. Normally **blood is supplied to the head by three routes**: through vessels in the ligamentum teres, through capsular vessels reflected onto the femoral neck, and through branches of nutrient vessels within the substance of the bone. When the fracture occurs, nutrient vessels are necessarily severed, capsular vessels are injured to varying degrees, and **blood supply is maintained only through the vessels in the ligamentum teres.** This is a variable quantity and is often insufficient, resulting in avascular necrosis of the femoral head.

ORTHOPEDIC

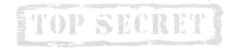

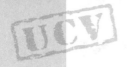
ID/CC

A **12-year-old obese male** is brought to the hospital with complaints of sudden-onset pain of the left hip along with a limp.

HPI

The pain is felt in the left groin and often radiates to the left thigh and knee.

PE

Left leg **externally rotated and about 2 cm shorter**; limited range of abduction and internal rotation; **upon flexing left hip, knee is drawn toward left axilla.**

Imaging

XR, left hip (AP view): **growth plate widened and irregular.**

Treatment

Single-screw fixation.

Discussion

Slipped femoral epiphyses affects youth 10 to 18 years old, with boys more commonly affected than girls; affected children may be overweight and in some cases have delayed sexual development. Represents a Salter-Harris type I epiphyseal injury. Twenty-five percent are bilateral, of which 15% to 20% occur simultaneously. **Avascular necrosis of the** femoral head and osteoarthritis may arise as complications.

hip – slipped capital femoral epiphyses

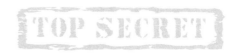

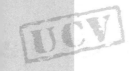

CASE 81

ID/CC
A 25-year-old female **athlete** is brought to the ER after she hurt her right knee.

HPI
She had **fallen on a hyperextended right knee** that has been unstable since the fall. She recalls having heard a "popping" sound at the time of the injury.

PE
Right knee exhibits effusion and **positive anterior "draw sign"** (tibia can be pulled forward on femur with knee flexed); instability of right knee joint (demonstrated by moving upper end of tibia forward on femur with knee flexed only 10 to 20 degrees [LACHMAN TEST]).

Imaging
MR, knee: indistinct, heterogenous signal in expected region of the anterior cruciate ligament.

Treatment
Surgical reconstruction for highly active patients; for less active patients, extensive physical therapy and avoidance of activity.

Discussion
The anterior cruciate ligament is torn by a force driving the upper end of the tibia forward relative to the femur or by hyperextension of the knee; the **posterior cruciate ligament is torn by a force driving the upper end of the tibia backward**.

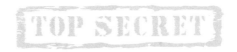

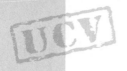

CASE 82

ID/CC
A 60-year-old **obese female** is seen with complaints of gradually pro gressing **stiffness and pain after use of the right knee.**

HPI
The pain and stiffness are accompanied by swelling and deformity of the joint. She also reports difficulty walking and limitation of movement.

PE
Tenderness, pain, and crepitus of right knee on motion; firm swelling (caused by underlying bony proliferations) and joint effusion; fixed deformities: bony enlargement and a varus angulation, causing limited motion at joint; hands show **bony swellings on distal interphalangeal joints** (HEBERDEN'S NODES).

Labs
Synovial fluid shows no evidence of inflammation; normal viscosity and mucin clot tests; protein, glucose, and complement levels also normal; serum rheumatoid factor not raised.

Imaging
XR, right knee (AP and lateral views): narrowing of joint space (medial > lateral); subchondral bone sclerosis; subchondral cysts and osteo phytes.

Gross Pathology
Late stages of the disease show **eburnation** of joint surface, **remodeling** of joint surface, **osteophytes** around lateral margins of joint, subchondral bone cysts, and bone sclerosis.

Micro Pathology
Loss of articular cartilage, bone resorption, and irregular and variable new bone and cartilage formation.

Treatment
Pain relief, improvement of mobility, and correction of deformity; joint replacement.

Discussion
Osteoarthritis, a degenerative joint disease, is characterized by the degeneration of articular cartilage and by progressive destruction and remodeling of the joint structures. The condition affects large weight bearing joints such as the knees, hips, and lumbar and cervical vertebrae; other joints commonly affected are the PIP, DIP, and first carpometa carpal joints. It is more common in women, and its incidence increases with age, particularly after 55.

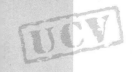

CASE 83

D/CC
A **12-year-old male** presents with a **swelling** above the right knee and associated pain.

HPI
There is **no history of trauma** at the site of pain. There has been **no discharge** from the swollen region and **no fever**.

PE
Bony-hard, tender, roughly circular swelling above right knee (**distal femur**); overlying skin temperature normal; mechanical restriction of movement of right knee.

Labs
Normal ESR; **elevated serum alkaline phosphatase** (may be used as marker of treatment response).

Imaging
XR, plain: osteoblastic bone lesion at distal end of femur with characteristic **"sunburst" or "onion-peel"** periosteal reaction; periosteal elevation by metaphyseal tumor (CODMAN'S TRIANGLE).

Gross Pathology
Firm, whitish mass with **osteoblastic** bone sclerosis originating from **metaphysis** adjacent to epiphyseal growth plate and invading through cortex, lifting up periosteum.

Micro Pathology
Bone biopsy shows multinucleated giant cells, anaplastic cells with pleomorphism, and osteoid production with foci of sarcomatous degeneration.

Treatment
Surgical amputation with total joint prosthesis or complex bone reconstruction; consider limb salvage; radiotherapy, chemotherapy.

Discussion
Osteogenic sarcoma is the most common primary malignant tumor of bone (excluding myeloma and lymphoma); it may be osteoblastic or osteolytic. Pathologic fractures may occur; pulmonary metastases are frequent. There is an increased risk with Paget's disease, prior radiation, and hereditary retinoblastoma.

ORTHOPEDIC

TOP SECRET

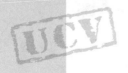

ID/CC

A 70-year-old male immigrant from England presents with **pain in the** right leg, producing an awkward gait, along with bilateral **hearing loss.**

HPI

He has also noted a progressive **increase in his hat size.**

PE

Slight **bowing of right tibia**; normal rectal exam; mixed conductive and **sensorineural hearing loss** confirmed by audiometry; physical exam otherwise normal.

Labs

Markedly elevated alkaline phosphatase; mildly elevated serum calcium and phosphorus; normal serum transaminases; **increased urinary excretion of hydroxyproline.**

Imaging

XR, skull: scattered **islands of bone lysis** (OSTEOPOROSIS CIRCUMSCRIPTA); mixed **thickening** (blastic) **and lucency** (lytic lesions) of bone (COTTON WOOL APPEARANCE). XR, leg (right side): bone soft with disorganized trabecular pattern; bowed tibia. XR, lumbar spine: enlargement of L vertebral body ("picture frame" pattern).

Gross Pathology

Expansion of bone cortex, blastic bone lesions, and bowing of long bone (thick ivory bones).

Micro Pathology

Multiple cement lines with unmineralized osteoid; indicative of excessive osteoblastic and osteoclastic activity.

Treatment

Medical treatment with bisphosphonates (inhibit osteoclastic activity), calcitonin; surgical treatment with total joint arthroplasty, nerve decompression, and osteotomies.

Discussion

A condition of probable viral etiology, Paget's disease is characterized by osteoclastic destruction of bone initially with excessive osteoblastic repair, producing bone sclerosis. When extensive, the resulting increased blood flow leads to **high cardiac output congestive heart failure.** Other complications are **pathologic fracture and osteosarcoma** (1% of patients).

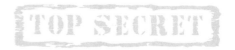

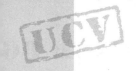
ID/CC   A **5-year-old male** is brought to a physician with sudden-onset progressive severe **pain, swelling, and redness** of the right knee joint.

HPI   He has had a **high-grade fever** for the past 2 days. A few days ago he **injured his right leg, and the injury subsequently became infected**; he is now unable to move his right leg properly.

PE   VS: fever. PE: infected wound on right leg; right **knee red, swollen, and tender**; all movements restricted by pain.

Labs   CBC: **neutrophilic leukocytosis** with shift to the left. Elevated ESR; synovial fluid (obtained following joint aspiration) opaque and yellowish; joint effusion has WBC count > 50,000/μL; Gram stain reveals **gram-positive cocci in clusters**; culture yields coagulase-positive *Staphylococcus aureus*.

Imaging   XR, right knee: early, soft tissue swelling and joint effusion; late, articular erosions and reactive sclerosis. NUC, gallium scan: increased uptake by right knee joint.

Treatment   **Broad-spectrum parenteral antibiotics** initially, then specific antibiotics following culture sensitivity reports; if necessary, joint may be opened, washed, and closed with a suction drain and immobilized until signs of inflammation subside.

Discussion   Septic arthritis is caused by pyogenic organisms and is more common among children, especially males. *S. aureus* is the most common cause; other organisms include streptococci, gonococci, pneumococci, and *Neisseria meningitidis*. Organisms reach the joint via hematogenous routes (most common; the primary focus may be a pyoderma, throat infection, IV drug use, etc.), secondary to adjacent osteomyelitis, or via penetrating wounds, or the condition may be iatrogenic.

ORTHOPEDIC

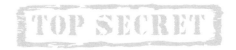

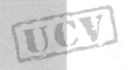

CASE 86

ID/CC   A 55-year-old woman presents with an **aching pain in the back of her neck**, a feeling of stiffness, and a "grating" sensation upon movement.

HPI   She also has a history of a vague, ill-defined, and ill-localized pain spreading over her shoulder region. She does not complain of any noticeable motor weakness or sensory loss over any part of the body and has no bladder or bowel complaints.

PE   Neck **slightly kyphotic; posterior cervical muscles tender; neck movements** slightly **restricted at extremes** due to pain; **audible crepitation on movement; diminished supinator and biceps reflex in the left upper limb**; no motor or sensory loss demonstrable.

Imaging   XR, cervical spine (lateral view): **narrowing of intervertebral disk space with formation of osteophytes at vertebral margins**, especially anteriorly.

Treatment   There is a strong tendency for the **symptoms of cervical spondylosis to subside spontaneously.** Treatment includes **analgesics, physiotherapy, and support of the neck** by a closely fitting collar of plaster or plastic. Surgical intervention is required for patients who are unresponsive to conservative therapy as well as for those with progressive myelopathy or radiculopathy.

Discussion   Degenerative arthritis occurs predominantly in the **lowest three cervical joints**. The changes **first affect the central intervertebral joints and later affect the posterior intervertebral (facet) joints. Osteophytes commonly encroach on the intervertebral foramina,** reducing the space for transmission of the cervical nerves. If the restricted space is further reduced by the traumatic edema of the contained soft tissues, manifestations of nerve pressure are likely to occur. Rarely, the spinal cord itself may suffer damage, producing a cervical myelopathy.

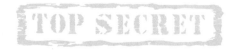

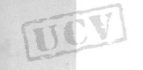

CASE 87

ID/CC   An asymptomatic **60-year-old** white **male** undergoing a routine physical exam is discovered to have a **pulsating abdominal mass**.

HPI   The patient has a history of **occasional abdominal pain** and **hyper-cholesterolemia** that has been poorly controlled by diet and medication.

PE   **Pulsating, painless upper abdominal mass** approximately 5 cm in diameter.

Imaging   KUB, lateral: calcification of aneurysm wall. CT/US, abdomen: dilated aorta with irregular calcified wall; large, eccentric mural thrombus seen.

Gross Pathology   Most aneurysms are located between renal arteries and iliac bifurcation; thrombus may also be present; intramural dissection may also be seen.

Micro Pathology   Aneurysm wall contains all three layers (intima, media, adventitia) ("TRUE" ANEURYSM).

Treatment   **Surgical replacement with graft** (if > 5.5 cm or symptomatic); consider endovascular stent/graft.

Discussion   The risk of rupture with potentially fatal bleeding increases with size. Abdominal aortic aneurysm is usually caused by **atherosclerotic disease** and is often associated with coronary artery disease. It may also be caused by trauma, infection (e.g., syphilis), **cystic medial degeneration**, and arteritis. Sequelae include rupture, embolization, infection, vascular occlusion secondary to thrombus formation, and compression of adjacent structures (e.g., ureters, vertebrae).

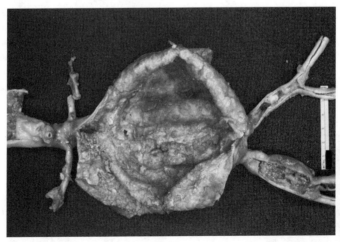

Figure 087 Large saccular swelling of the abdominal aorta just proximal to iliac bifurcation.

GENERAL SURGERY

87

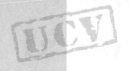

ID/CC
A 42-year-old white female, the mother of five, develops acute intermittent pain in the right upper quadrant and right scapula after eating a fatty meal.

HPI
She is of Native American ancestry and is 30 pounds overweight. She also complains of nausea and has vomited three times. She has had several prior episodes of similar pain following meals.

PE
VS: fever; tachycardia. PE: obese; tenderness in right upper abdominal quadrant with inspiratory arrest on palpation (MURPHY'S SIGN); hypoactive bowel sounds.

Labs
Hypercholesterolemia. CBC: leukocytosis with mild neutrophilia. Elevated direct bilirubin; elevated alkaline phosphatase.

Imaging
US: distended gallbladder with wall thickening containing multiple echogenic shadows (stones). Nuc, HIDA: failure to visualize gallbladder indicates cystic duct obstruction by stone.

Gross Pathology
Gallbladder inflammation ranging from wall edema to acute gangrene with necrosis, pus formation, and perforation with peritonitis. Most stones are composed of cholesterol; less common are pigmented stones made principally of unconjugated bilirubin and calcium salts.

Micro Pathology
Gallbladder mucosa contains lipid-laden foamy macrophages.

Treatment
Initial conservative treatment with IV fluids, analgesics, and antibiotics followed by elective cholecystectomy (usually laparoscopic) is definitive.

Discussion
Although calculi are involved in most cases of acute cholecystitis, acalculous cases arise after nonbiliary major surgeries, severe trauma or burns, and sepsis and in the postpartum state. Differential diagnosis includes appendicitis, pancreatitis, perforated peptic ulcer, pyelonephritis, myocardial infarction, and right lower lobe pneumonia. Clinical risk factors include the four F's: fat, female, forty, and fertile.

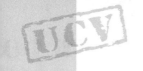

CASE 89

ID/CC A 17-year-old male student presents with **anorexia** and poorly localized **periumbilical pain** followed by **nausea** and two episodes of **vomiting**.

HPI Four hours after presentation, the **pain shifted to the right lower quadrant** and he developed a **low-grade fever**.

PE VS: mild tachycardia; low-grade fever. PE: **right lower quadrant tenderness with guarding and rebound**; pain in right lower quadrant when pressure applied to left lower quadrant (ROVSING'S SIGN); **pain localized to junction of outer and middle third of the line from anterior superior iliac spine to umbilicus** (MCBURNEY'S POINT); right lower quadrant pain elicited by passive hip flexion (PSOAS SIGN) and by passive internal and external rotation of hip (OBTURATOR SIGN).

Labs CBC: elevated WBC count; predominance of neutrophils. Normal serum amylase. UA: normal.

Imaging KUB: right psoas shadow blurred; generalized ileus with air-fluid levels; increased soft tissue density in right lower quadrant; small radiopaque fecalith in right lower quadrant. US: **noncompressible tubular structure** in right lower quadrant. CT, abdomen: enlarged appendix with enhancement of appendiceal wall and periappendiceal fat stranding.

Gross Pathology Early lesion: hyperemic appendix with fibrinous exudate; late lesion: purulent exudate with necrosis and perforation; fecalith occasionally present.

Treatment **Appendectomy** with preoperative antibiotic coverage.

Discussion The peak incidence of appendicitis is in the second and third decades. Causes include **obstruction by fecaliths** (33%) and **lymphoid hyperplasia** (60%); it is occasionally caused by tumors (carcinoid tumor is the most common tumor of the appendix), parasites, foreign bodies, and Crohn's disease. Complications include perforation, **periappendiceal abscess**, peritonitis, and generalized or wound sepsis.

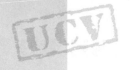

CASE 90

ID/CC	A **67-year-old** white female complains of increasing fatigue for several months.
HPI	She has also noticed significant **weight loss** and **intermittent diarrhea**.
PE	Marked **pallor**; palpable left supraclavicular lymph node (VIRCHOW'S NODE); palpable mass in right iliac fossa; hepatomegaly.
Labs	CBC/PBS: microcytic, hypochromic **anemia**. **Positive stool guaiac test**; elevated serum carcinoembryonic antigen (CEA) levels.
Imaging	BE: large, irregular fungating mass in cecum. US: metastatic hepatic nodules. Colonoscopy: large fungating growth in cecum.
Gross Pathology	Cauliflower-like, **fungating, nonobstructing growth** in cecum; may be polypoid, sessile, or constricting.
Micro Pathology	Well-differentiated **adenocarcinoma**.
Treatment	Right hemicolectomy with regional lymph node dissection for staging; adjuvant chemotherapy in selected patients; follow up for recurrence by monitoring CEA levels.
Discussion	Starting at age 50, colon cancer screening with colonoscopy and fecal occult blood testing is recommended for the average-risk population.

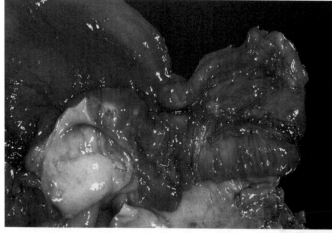

Figure 090 Fungating mass replacing the cecal wall and constricting the lumen.

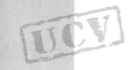
ID/CC A 68-year-old **black male** presents with anorexia, progressive **dysphagia**, odynophagia, and **weight loss**.

HPI The patient has been drinking very **hot tea** since he was 11 years old and **smokes** one pack of cigarettes per day. His history also reveals heavy **alcohol** intake; occasional cough, vomiting, and **regurgitation**; and severe dysphagia with **solids, progressing to liquids**.

PE Emaciation; fixed, **nonpainful supraclavicular node**; pale conjunctiva.

Labs CBC/PBS: hypochromic, microcytic anemia. Hemoccult-positive stool; hypoalbuminemia.

Imaging UGI: **irregular fungating esophageal mass** in middle third of esophagus with partial obstruction. CT, chest: irregular esophageal mass with invasion of mediastinum and enlarged para-aortic lymph node.

Gross Pathology Large fungating mass protruding toward esophageal lumen.

Micro Pathology Squamous cell carcinoma on biopsy.

Treatment Laser ablation of tumor with palliative stent placement; palliative radiotherapy; surgical resection followed by chemotherapy plus radiotherapy for curable tumors; eventual gastrostomy tube placement.

Discussion The most common variant of esophageal carcinoma is **squamous cell carcinoma (SCC)**, which is associated with alcohol and tobacco use and is more common in blacks. Although the incidence of SCC is decreasing in the United States, the incidence of adenocarcinoma is rising dramatically and is more common in whites with **Barrett's syndrome** (glandular metaplasia of the squamous epithelium of the distal esophagus is caused by chronic, untreated gastroesophageal reflux disease).

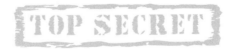

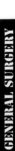

GENERAL SURGERY

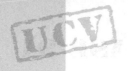
ID/CC   An 83-year-old white male complains of **anorexia, frequent vomiting** and a **gnawing midepigastric pain** of several months' duration.

HPI   The pain is **not relieved by antacids or milk**. The patient has lost **significant weight** over the past few months due to diarrhea after every meal.

PE   Pale, **emaciated** male in moderate distress; left supraclavicular lymph node (VIRCHOW'S NODE) palpable.

Labs   CBC: **hypochromic, microcytic anemia**. Stool **positive for occult blood** LFTs normal.

Imaging   UGI: large fungating lesion on greater curvature of stomach with fistulous tract running to transverse colon. EGD: same.

Gross Pathology   Polyploid, raised, fungating mass projecting into lumen; situated at distal end of stomach.

Micro Pathology   Biopsy reveals a **well-differentiated adenocarcinoma** with **signet-ring** cells.

Treatment   Esophagogastrectomy for tumors of the cardia and gastroesophageal junction; subtotal gastrectomy for tumors of the distal stomach; radiotherapy; chemotherapy.

Discussion   Most commonly found on the **lesser curvature** in the **antrum** and pyloric areas, adenocarcinomas may be one of two types: **intestinal** and **diffuse**. Chronic atrophic gastritis, pernicious anemia, infection with *H. pylori*, postsurgical gastric remnants, and type A blood are all predisposing risk factors for the development of adenocarcinoma. It most commonly spreads hematogenously to the liver and may spread transperitoneally to the ovaries (KRUKENBERG TUMOR).

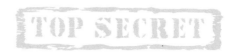

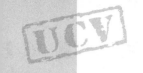

CASE 93

ID/CC	A 44-year-old male is admitted to the hospital following episodes of **vomiting blood** (HEMATEMESIS) and passing **black, tarry, foul-smelling stools** (MELENA).
HPI	He has experienced **recurrent painless hematemesis** and **melena** for several years, but repeated evaluations have been negative.
PE	Pallor.
Labs	CBC: **microcytic, hypochromic anemia**. Nasogastric aspirate has **coffee-ground** appearance.
Imaging	UGI/EGD: 5-cm mass in fundus of stomach with 2-cm ulcer on surface.
Gross Pathology	Postoperative specimen reveals a firm, circumscribed nodular **mass within the gastric wall** covered by mucosa.
Micro Pathology	Whorling interlaced bundles of spindle-shaped cells; no evidence of anaplasia.
Treatment	Surgical resection.
Discussion	Gastric leiomyoma is the **most common benign** tumor of the **stomach**.

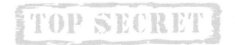

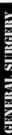

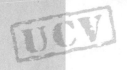

ID/CC   A 40-year-old male presents with **cramping abdominal pain** and **vomiting** of 3 hours' duration.

HPI   He also complains of an **inability to pass stool or flatus** (OBSTIPATION) for the past 3 days. Two years ago, he underwent an emergency appendectomy for a ruptured appendix.

PE   Dehydration; **abdominal distention**; generalized mild tenderness over abdomen without rebound or guarding; bowel sounds heard as **high-pitched tinkles during pain paroxysms**; empty rectal vault on rectal exam.

Labs   CBC/PBS: leukocytosis with hemoconcentration. Serum amylase levels normal.

Imaging   XR, abdomen: "stepladder" pattern of multiple **dilated loops of small bowel** and **multiple air-fluid levels**; **colon and rectum gasless** (air in colon or rectum would indicate an intestinal ileus); no free air under diaphragm.

Treatment IV fluid and electrolyte replacement; nasogastric suction/decompression; broad-spectrum antibiotics; surgery.

Discussion The most common causes of small bowel obstruction are intestinal **adhesions secondary to prior abdominal surgery, intussusception, volvulus,** and **incarcerated hernia**; the most common causes of large bowel obstruction are **carcinoma, volvulus,** and **sigmoid diverticulitis.** Complications include **strangulation** and **necrosis** of the bowel wall leading to perforation, peritonitis, sepsis, and shock.

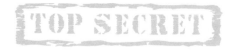

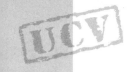
ID/CC   An **18-month-old male** is brought to the emergency room by his parents because of acute, **intermittent abdominal pain**, abdominal distention, and passage of "**red currant jelly**" **stools**.

HPI   The child had previously been well, and his immunization schedule is complete. He **vomited** twice following admission.

PE   Child crying and screaming, with knees drawn to abdomen; abdomen tender and distended; **oblong** (sausage-shaped) **mass** in abdomen (most often in right upper quadrant) that hardens with palpation; examining finger stained with **mucus and blood** on digital rectal examination.

Labs   No parasites on stool exam; no pathogen on stool culture.

Imaging   XR, abdomen: gas in small intestine and absence of cecal gas shadow. BE: **telescoping** of ileum into cecum.

Gross Pathology   During operation, three layers are seen: entering or inner tube, returning or middle tube, and sheath or outer tube; outer tube called intussuscipiens; inner and middle together called intussusceptum.

Micro Pathology   **Ischemic necrosis** with sloughing of mucosa, producing "red currant jelly" stools.

Treatment   Hydrostatic (barium) or pneumatic (air) **reduction** using an enema; surgical reduction or resection if that fails or is contraindicated owing to perforation or gangrene.

Discussion   Ninety-five percent of cases of intussusception are idiopathic and usually originate near the ileocecal junction. The condition is associated with adenovirus infections, which produce **hyperplasia of Peyer's patches** in the terminal ileum, which serves as a nidus for intussusception. It is also seen with **lead points** (e.g., Meckel's diverticulum, polyps, parasites, duplications, hemangiomas, and suture lines).

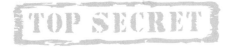

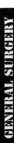

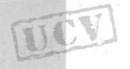

ID/CC A 51-year-old male complains of **pruritus** and **abdominal pain** that radiates to his back along with **significant weight loss** (15 kg) over the past 4 months.

HPI He also states that his **urine is dark** and that his **stools are clay-colored** (ACHOLIC). He admits to a history of **smoking** (60 pack-years) and heavy alcohol use with **multiple prior bouts of pancreatitis**.

PE Cachectic male; **scleral icterus** (indicates jaundice); **hepatomegaly**; **palpable gallbladder** (COURVOISIER'S SIGN); hard 8-cm mass palpable in **midepigastric** region.

Labs Markedly elevated direct bilirubin (20 mg/dL); absence of urinary urobilinogen; markedly **elevated alkaline phosphatase**; mildly elevated transaminases; normal PT; **elevated carcinoembryonic antigen (CEA) and CA 19-9**.

Imaging CT/US: **mass in head of pancreas; dilated intrahepatic bile ducts**. ERCP: abrupt cutoff of main pancreatic duct. UGI: narrowed lumen of duodenum.

Gross Pathology Hard nodular mass with ill-defined borders invading pancreatic parenchyma and **obstructing common bile duct** around head of pancreas with local extension and liver metastases.

Micro Pathology Pancreatic mass biopsy reveals a poorly differentiated **ductal adenocarcinoma** in clusters, secreting mucin and dense collagenous desmoplastic stroma.

Treatment Surgical pancreaticoduodenectomy (WHIPPLE'S PROCEDURE); chemotherapy; supportive and palliative care (biliary decompression to relieve jaundice; celiac plexus block for pain).

Discussion Chronic gallbladder disease, diabetes mellitus, hereditary pancreatitis, **chronic pancreatitis, cigarette smoking**, diets high in meat and fat, and occupational exposure to **carcinogens** are predisposing factors. Pancreatic carcinoma carries a **poor prognosis** (85% are already locally invasive or metastatic at the time of diagnosis) and is associated with a mutation in the K-ras oncogene and the p53 tumor suppressor gene. Complications include hypercoagulability (resulting in **migratory thrombophlebitis**, also known as the Trousseau sign).

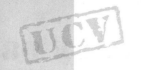
ID/CC
A term female newborn is noted to have **edema, dyspnea, cyanosis, and marked jaundice**.

HPI
Her **mother is blood type** AB **Rh-negative**. Her **previous childbirth** was an uneventful full-term vaginal delivery conducted outside the United States 4 years ago. The mother **did not receive any subsequent immunizations**.

PE
Pallor; **marked jaundice**; hypotonia; **S3 and S4**; hepatosplenomegaly; **generalized edema**.

Labs
Blood type of **mother AB Rh negative**; blood type of father A Rh positive; **blood type of first child A Rh positive**. Mother's serum: **positive indirect Coombs' test**, anti-D antibody titer > 1:64. Neonate's serum: positive direct Coombs' test, increased indirect bilirubin.

Gross Pathology
Brain specimen from autopsy reveals yellow staining of basal ganglia by unconjugated bilirubin (KERNICTERUS).

Treatment
Phototherapy (promotes elimination of bilirubin); exchange transfusion.

Discussion
The mother produced anti-D (IgG) antibodies owing to her exposure to D antigen during her delivery of an Rh-positive infant. In her subsequent pregnancy, these antibodies crossed the placenta and reacted with the fetus's RBCs (Rh positive), producing hemolysis and fetal heart failure with generalized edema (HYDROPS FETALIS). To prevent Rh isoimmunization, all Rh-negative mothers with an Rh-positive fetus should receive RhO (D) immune globulin following deliveries, abortions, ectopic pregnancies, or even amniocentesis.

erythroblastosis fetalis

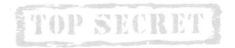

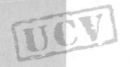

ID/CC   Paramedics are called at 7:00 AM because a **2-month-old male**, the child of African immigrants, cannot be awakened by his mother; upon arrival, it is clear that the child has been dead for at least 4 hours.

HPI   The child was slightly premature, but aside from this, his history was unremarkable. There was nothing that could directly explain the episode. On directed history, **the mother admits to being a smoker and remembers that the child had a URI 4 days ago.**

PE   No pathologic cause revealed that could explain death.

Gross Pathology Autopsy reveals petechiae on pleural and pericardial surfaces, pulmonary congestion, and scattered foci of lymphocytic tissue in interstitium of lungs.

Discussion   Sudden infant death syndrome (SIDS) refers to **death of an infant under 1 year of age**, usually during sleep, in which **death remains unexplained** even after complete autopsy; most have a **history of minor URIs.**

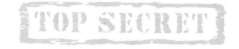

ANSWER KEY

1. Aortic Dissection
2. Aortic Insufficiency
3. Aortic Stenosis
4. Atherosclerosis
5. Atrial Fibrillation
6. Atrial Myxoma
7. CAD—Myocardial Infarction
8. Cardiac Tamponade
9. Cardiac Transplant
10. Congestive Heart Failure
11. Constrictive Pericarditis
12. Cor Pulmonale
13. Dilated Cardiomyopathy
14. Eisenmenger's Complex
15. High-Altitude Sickness
16. Hypertrophic Obstructive Cardiomyopathy
17. Hypothermia
18. Malignant Hypertension
19. Marantic Endocarditis
20. Mitral Insufficiency
21. Mitral Stenosis
22. Myocarditis
23. Peripheral Arterial Embolism
24. Shock—Hypovolemic
25. Sinus Bradycardia
26. Syphilis—Tertiary (Aortitis)
27. Thromboangiitis Obliterans (Buerger's Disease)
28. Thrombophlebitis—Superficial
29. Wolff–Parkinson–White Syndrome
30. Actinic Keratosis
31. Atopic Dermatitis
32. Basal Cell Carcinoma
33. Contact Dermatitis
34. Dermatitis Herpetiformis
35. Dysplastic Nevus Syndrome
36. Erythema Multiforme
37. Furuncle
38. Kaposi's Sarcoma
39. Kawasaki's Syndrome
40. Lichen Planus
41. Malignant Melanoma
42. Mycosis Fungoides
43. Osler–Weber–Rendu Syndrome
44. Pemphigus
45. Pityriasis Rosea
46. Psoriasis
47. Pyoderma Gangrenosum
48. Seborrheic Dermatitis
49. Serum Sickness
50. Vitiligo
51. Acute Tubular Necrosis (ATN)
52. Adult Polycystic Kidney Disease (APKD)
53. Alport's Disease
54. Amyloidosis—Primary
55. Benign Prostatic Hypertrophy (BPH)
56. Bladder Cancer
57. Bladder Outlet Obstruction, Nephropathy
58. Diabetic Nephropathy
59. Goodpasture's Syndrome
60. Hypertensive Renal Disease
61. IgA Nephropathy (Berger's Disease)
62. Lupus Nephritis
63. Membranoproliferative Glomerulonephritis (MPGN)
64. Membranous Glomerulonephritis
65. Minimal Change Disease
66. Prostate Carcinoma
67. Renal Cell Carcinoma
68. Renal Infarction
69. Renovascular Hypertension
70. Seminoma
71. Testicular Choriocarcinoma
72. Testicular Dysgenesis
73. Testicular Teratoma (Mixed)
74. Testicular Torsion
75. Urate Nephropathy
76. Wilms' Tumor
77. Ewing's Sarcoma
78. Hand—Dupuytren's Contracture
79. Hip—Avascular Necrosis of Femoral Head
80. Hip—Slipped Capital Femoral Epiphysis
81. Knee—Anterior Cruciate Ligament Injury
82. Osteoarthritis
83. Osteogenic Sarcoma
84. Paget's Disease of Bone

85. Septic Arthritis—Staphylococcal

86. Spine—Cervical Spondylosis

87. Abdominal Aortic Aneurysm

88. Acute Cholecystitis

89. Appendicitis

90. Cecal Carcinoma

91. Esophageal Carcinoma

92. Gastric Carcinoma

93. Gastric Leiomyoma

94. Intestinal Obstruction—Acute

95. Intussusception

96. Pancreatic Carcinoma

97. Erythroblastosis Fetalis

98. Sudden Infant Death Syndrome (SIDS)

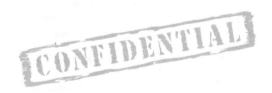

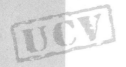
1. A 28-year-old white female presents with a diffuse rash. The rash involves hair follicles, with apparent pustules. The patient reports a history of recent hot tub use. What are the characteristic findings regarding the responsible bacterium?

   A: Colorless colonies on MacConkey agar; oxidase positive; blue-green-pigment on nutrient agar.

   B: Colorless colonies on MacConkey agar; urease positive; blackens triple sugar iron agar.

   C: Colorless colonies on MacConkey agar; oxidase negative; no gas on triple sugar iron agar.

   D: Colored (pink) colonies on MacConkey agar; urease positive.

   E: Colored (pink) colonies on MacConkey agar; metallic green sheen on EMB agar.

2. A 24-year-old male is thrown from a car that he drove into a tree. He suffers from a T6 spinal crush injury. After he recovers from his acute injury, what is the most appropriate course of action regarding his bladder?

   A: The patient should be taught how to self-catherize himself, because he will never be able to control his bladder.

   B: The patient will have a bladder that fills and dribbles urine all the time.

   C: The bladder is paralyzed and the patient will have to use abdominal compression and straining to void.

   D: The bladder should remain catherized until micturation reflexes return. The patient can then be taught to cutaneously stimulate the genital area to stimulate a micturation reflex.

   E: The patient will have frequent bladder reflux with resulting bladder infections.

3. A 78-year-old frail appearing white female presents to clinic for a physical. She has no complaints or concerns. Past medical history is significant for hypertension as well as a fractured left hip 3 years ago after a fall. The patient is takes atenolol and a multivitamin. She smokes 1 pack of cigarettes per day, denies alcohol and drug use. Physical exam reveals no gross abnormalities. A bone scan is ordered and shows that her bone density is 2.5 standard deviations below the mean for her age. Which of the following lab abnormalities might you expect in this patient?

   A: Decreased calcium, increased phosphate, normal alkaline phosphatase

   B: Normal calcium, normal phosphate, increased alkaline phosphatase

   C: Increased calcium, decreased phosphate, increased alkaline phosphatase

   D: Increased calcium, increased phosphate, normal alkaline phosphatase

   E: Normal calcium, normal phosphate, normal alkaline phosphatase

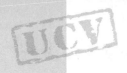

4. You are on a surgical rotation and 3 days ago you got to close the incision on the "big" surgery that took 10 hours. On attending rounds you are asked the following question: "If we were to biopsy your perfectly closed and healing wound what would we expect to find?"

    A: Granulation tissue, a great amount of neovascularization, evidence of epithelial proliferation
    B: The incision filled with clot
    C: Macrophages and granulation tissue
    D: Neutrophils, mitoses in the epithelial basal cells and closure of the wound site
    E: Proliferation of fibroblasts, a great amount of collagen deposition enough to produce a small scar, no inflammation or newly formed vessels

5. You are working in a busy urology clinic and see a patient that was just sent up from the ER. He is complaining of pain in his back from which he cannot get comfortable. He was diagnosed with a stone before by finding it in his urine. Today he has blood in his urine but an abdominal x-ray without contrast shows no evidence of stone, but he does have blood in his urine. His stone is likely made of which of the following?

    A: Ammonium, magnesium, and phosphate
    B: Calcium
    C: Cystine
    D: Phosphate
    E: Uric acid

6. Prior to beginning your nephrology rotation, you decide to review nephron physiology. Which of the following is a true statement regarding the nephron?

    A: Early distal convoluted tubule actively reabsorbs both sodium and chloride
    B: Early distal convoluted tubule passively reabsorbs water
    C: The thin descending loop of Henle actively reabsorbs potassium, chloride, and sodium
    D: The thick ascending loop of Henle passively reabsorbs water
    E: The thick ascending loop of Henle reabsorbs all of the glucose and amino acids

7. A 23-year-old man is in a car accident. The man receives a significant abdominal laceration that results in 1-liter blood loss. The trauma surgeon is able to ligate the bleeding artery and stop further bleeding. A hypertonic fluid is given through an IV line. What changes would you expect to occur to extracellular fluid volume, body osmolarity, and intercellular fluid volume respectively due to the hypertonic fluid?

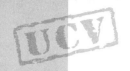
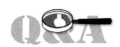

A: Decrease, increase, decrease
B: Decrease, no change, no change
C: Increase, decrease, increase
D: Increase, increase, decrease
E: Increase, no change, no change

8. Your 72-year-old patient presented to your office with severe back pain, upper leg pain, hearing loss, and high some signs of cardiac failure. You took an x-ray of the pelvis and noticed that bone architecture in the femur and spine was abnormal. You described the architecture as "mosaic." Which lab abnormalities would you expect to see in this patient?

A: Increased alkaline phosphatase levels
B: Decreased calcium levels
C: Decreased phosphorus levels
D: Decreased alkaline phosphatase levels
E: Normal alkaline phosphatase levels

9. The most common cause of chronic cor pulmonale is which of the following?

A: Asthma
B: Chronic increased oxygen saturation
C: Left-sided heart failure
D: Myocardial infarction
E: Pulmonary embolism

10. A 76-year-old man comes to the clinic complaining of shortness of breath for the last month. Physical exam reveals a systolic murmur that radiates the axilla. The physician decides to order an echocardiogram to confirm his diagnosis. What statement is correct regarding valvular problems?

A: Aortic stenosis results in eccentric hypertrophy of the left ventricle.
B: Mitral regurgitation is associated with a murmur that radiates to the neck.
C: Mitral regurgitation usually results in a systolic apical murmur that may radiate to the axilla.
D: Mitral stenosis results in a systolic murmur.
E: Pulmonic stenosis results in pulmonary edema.

11. A 28-year-old patient with a history of multiple fractures and recent-onset fatigue is referred to your medical center from the community for further work-up. During the evaluation process, the patient begins to complain of difficulty with his vision. The best explanation for this presentation is:

A: Osteopetrosis
B: Temporal arteritis
C: Alport's syndrome
D: Diabetes mellitus
E: Iron deficiency anemia

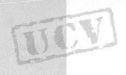

12. A 35-year-old female patient comes to your office with complaints of palpitations and light-headedness. After an extensive cardiac workup reveals no definitive abnormalities, you learn that such "spells" are extremely common in her family. Genetic testing reveals that she has a mutation in the delayed rectifier potassium channel that decreases its conductance. Which one of the following best represents the effects of this mutation in ventricular myocyte action potentials?

   A: Reduced overshoot of the action potential
   B: Reduced duration of the plateau of the action potenial
   C: Prolonged phase 1 repolarization
   D: Prolonged plateau due to prolongation of phase 2
   E: Less negative resting potential

13. A 76-year-old female is complaining of urine leakage when coughing and standing up. The problem has gotten worse after her hysterectomy about 1 month ago for suspected endometrial cancer. Urine culture is negative for significant bacteria. What is the next appropriate pharmacologic step?

   A: Alpha 1 agonist
   B: Alpha 2 antagonist
   C: Beta 2 antagonist
   D: Beta 1 agonist
   E: Muscarinic agonist

14. Your 60-year-old female patient has been suffering from osteoporosis for 5 years now. Recently, she also developed mild hypertension. You decide that it is appropriate to start treating her with a diuretic. The most appropriate diuretic is:

   A: Acetazolamide
   B: Amiloride
   C: Clorothiazide
   D: Furosemide
   E: Mannitol

15. A 78-year-old frail appearing white female presents to clinic for a physical. She has no complaints or concerns. Past medical history is significant for hypertension as well as a fractured left hip 3 years ago after a fall. The patient is takes atenolol and a multivitamin. She smokes one pack of cigarettes per day, denies alcohol and drug use. Physical exam reveals no gross abnormalities. A bone scan is ordered and shows that her bone density is 2.5 standard deviations below the mean for her age. Which of the following lab abnormalities might you expect in this patient?

   A: Decreased calcium, increased phosphate, normal alkaline phosphatase
   B: Normal calcium, normal phosphate, increased alkaline phosphatase

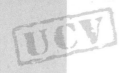
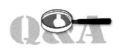

C: Increased calcium, decreased phosphate, increased alkaline phosphatase

D: Increased calcium, increased phosphate, normal alkaline phosphatase

E: Normal calcium normal phosphate, normal alkaline phosphatase

16. A 17-year-old Honduran male presents to your office, because of increasing spells of losing attention and falling during exercise. He has also noted feeling some shortness of breath lately. The patient states that he has always had these spells, but previously they happened rarely. On further questioning you find out that a brother, father, paternal aunt, and grandmother all had similar spells. The patient has another brother who is unaffected. The brother who had these spells died when he was 14. One of his father's siblings who did not have these spells died suddenly at age 18 during a soccer game. On physical examination, you would expect to hear which of the following cardiac murmurs:

   A: A continuous murmur.

   B: A crescendo-decrescendo systolic ejection murmur beginning immediately after S_1.

   C: A crescendo-decrescendo systolic ejection murmur beginning well after S_1.

   D: High pitched diastolic murmur beginning immediately after S_2.

   E: High pitched systolic murmur beginning well after S_2, often accompanied with an initial snap.

17. A 62-year-old man with diabetes and chronic renal failure is given vitamin D supplementation. Why was this done?

   A: Inability for the activated vitamin D to bind to the cytosolic receptor in the intestine.

   B: Inability to create 7-dehydrocholesterol. 1 hydroxylase.

   C: Inability to make 25-hydroxy 1 hydroxylase.

   D: Inability to make more calcium binding protein once activated vitamin D has changed transcription.

   E: Inability to make cholecalciferol.

18. A 55-year-old alcoholic patient presents to cardiology after having an ECHO that revealed dilated congestive heart failure. No other abnormalities are noted. Which of the following abnormal physical exam findings might you expect?

   A: S_1

   B: S_2

   C: S_3

   D: S_4

   E: Jugular venous distention

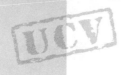

19. A 76-year-old white female presents to the family practice clinic with the complaint of lesion on her forehead. History reveals that she has farmed tobacco for the majority of her adult life. She reports that the lesion seems to be expanding. The papule measures 8 mm, and appears to be pearly, almost translucent, with telangiectasias. What will the pathology report reveal?

A: Sheets of neoplastic cells with keratin pearls
B: Central connective tissue core under squamous epithelium
C: Vacuolated cells in the epidermis granular layer
D: Intertwining bundles of collagen and fibroblasts
E: Palisading clusters of darkly staining cells

20. A 6-month-old child is being evaluated for a ventricular septal defect. Which of the following murmurs would you most expect on physical exam?

A: Continuous machine-like murmur
B: Crescendo-decrescendo systolic ejection murmur
C: Holosystolic murmur
D: Late diastolic murmur
E: Systolic murmur with a midsystolic click

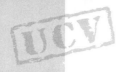

ANSWERS

1. A

    A: Colorless colonies on MacConkey agar; oxidase positive; blue-green-pigment on nutrient agar. [Correct] *Pseudomonas aeruginosa* causes pneumonia, urinary tract infections, sepsis, and hot tub folliculitis. *Pseudomonas* grows in water, and can withstand many detergents and disinfectants. Pyocyanin gene product gives purulent material a bluish hue, while pyoverdin is seen as yellow-green with ultraviolet light. Ultraviolet light may be used to assess cutaneous infection by *Pseudomonas* in burn patients. *Pseudomonas* does not ferment glucose.

    B: Colorless colonies on MacConkey agar; urease positive; blackens triple sugar iron agar. [Incorrect] Proteus commonly causes urinary tract infections. Liberation of ammonia by urease increases urine pH, which increases the potential for struvite stone development.

    C: Colorless colonies on MacConkey agar; oxidase negative; no gas on triple sugar iron agar. [Incorrect] *Shigella* is characterized by its virulence—only 100 bacteria must be ingested to develop shigellosis. Person-to-person acquisition is common, via fingers, flies, food, and feces. Symptoms begin as fever and abdominal pain, progressing to watery diarrhea, which later consists of blood and mucus. No rash is associated with shigellosis. Lactose is not fermented, as evidenced by colorless colonies on MacConkey agar.

    D: Colored (pink) colonies on MacConkey agar; urease positive. [Incorrect] *Klebsiella* is found in the large intestine, soil sources, and water sources. The thick capsule is characteristic of this bacterium. *Klebsiella* causes pneumonia in the elderly, diabetic patients, patients with chronic obstructive pulmonary disease, and alcoholics. Pink coloration on MacConkey plates indicates lactose fermentation. Current jelly sputum, necrosis, and abscess formation are commonly associated with pneumonia caused by *Klebsiella*.

    E: Colored (pink) colonies on MacConkey agar; metallic green sheen on EMB agar. [Incorrect] *Escherichia coli* causes diarrhea, urinary tract infections, hemolytic-uremic.

2. D

    A: The patient should be taught how to self-catherize himself, because he will never be able to control his bladder. [Incorrect] Self-catherization is appropriate if the patient can never control his bladder. This can be caused by loss of sensory nerves.

    B: The patient will have a bladder that fills and dribbles urine all the time. [Incorrect] Lesions that affect the sensory nerves prevent normal micturation reflex. The bladder will fill to capacity and overflow a little at a time.

    C: The bladder is paralyzed and the patient will have to use abdominal compression and straining to void. [Incorrect] Bladder paralysis will

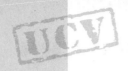

be caused by lesions below T12. Abdominal straining and compression, called Crede's manuver, will often allow voiding.

D: The bladder should remain catherized until micturation reflexes return. The patient can then be taught to cutaneously stimulate the genital area to stimulate a micturation reflex. [Correct] Here spinal shock causes complete suppression of the micturation reflex for the first few days.

E: The patient will have frequent bladder reflux with resulting bladder infections. [Incorrect] Bladder dyssynergia can be caused by upper spinal cord lesions. This causes ureteral reflux.

3.   E

A: Decreased calcium, increased phosphate, normal alkaline phosphatase [Incorrect] The above patient has osteoporosis. A patient with decreased calcium, increased phosphate, and normal alkaline phosphatase would most likely present with renal insufficiency.

B: Normal calcium, normal phosphate, increased alkaline phosphatase [Incorrect] A patient with normal calcium, normal phosphate, and increased alkaline phosphatase would not suggest osteoporosis.

C: Increased calcium, decreased phosphate, increased alkaline phosphatase [Incorrect] A patient with increased calcium, decreased phosphate, and increased alkaline phosphatase would not have osteoporosis. This patient could be a candidate for hyperparathyroidism.

D: Increased calcium, increased phosphate, normal alkaline phosphatase [Incorrect] These labs would not suggest osteoporosis. It could however, suggest Vitamin D intoxication.

E: Normal calcium, normal phosphate, normal alkaline phosphatase [Correct] The patient most likely has osteoporosis; therefore, her calcium, phosphate, and alkaline phosphatase would most likely be normal.

4.   C

A: Granulation tissue, a great amount of neovascularization, evidence of epithelial proliferation [Incorrect] This is typically seen at day 5

B: The incision filled with clot [Incorrect] This is typically found for only a few hours after primary closure of the wound.

C: Macrophages and granulation tissue [Correct] This is typical for day 3.

D: Neutrophils, mitoses in the epithelial basal cells and closure of the wound site [Incorrect] This stage is typically seen 3–24 hours after closure.

E: Proliferation of fibroblasts, a great amount of collagen deposition enough to produce a small scar, no inflammation or newly formed vessels [Incorrect] This stage is found after 2 weeks of healing.

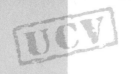

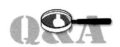

5.   E

A: Ammonium, magnesium, and phosphate [Incorrect] Also known as staghorn or struvite stones which can form large stony structures that will not pass. These stones are usually associated with infections with ammonia producing organisms such as *Proteus vulgaris* and *Staphylococcus*. These are visible by x-ray.

B: Calcium [Incorrect] These stones are very visible on x-ray and account for 80–85% of stones.

C: Cystine [Incorrect] Almost always associated with cystinuria and visible by x-ray.

D: Phosphate [Incorrect] Sometimes refers to staghorn calculi.

E: Uric acid [Correct] Uric acid is <u>U</u>nseen on x-ray.

6.   A

A: Early distal convoluted tubule actively reabsorbs both sodium and chloride [Correct] The early distal convoluted tubule is responsible for actively reabsorbing both sodium and chloride.

B: Early distal convoluted tubule passively reabsorbs water [Incorrect] The early distal convoluted tubule is responsible for actively reabsorbing both sodium and choloride.

C: The thin descending loop of Henle actively reabsorbs potassium, chloride, and sodium [Incorrect] The thin descending loop of Henle is responsible for the passive reabsorption of water.

D: The thick ascending loop of Henle passively reabsorbs water [Incorrect] The thick ascending loop of Henle is responsible for the active reabsorption of sodium, chloride, and potassium. Water does not pass through its membrane.

E: The thick ascending loop of Henle reabsorbs all of the glucose and amino acids [Incorrect] As mentioned above the thick ascending loop of Henle actively reabsorbs potassium, chloride, and sodium. The early proximal convoluted tubule reabsorbs all of the glucose and amino acids.

7.   D

A: Decrease, increase, decrease [Incorrect] This pattern is more consistent with loss of hypotonic fluid such as in dehydration, diabetes insipidus, and alcoholism.

B: Decrease, no change, no change [Incorrect] This is pattern is more consistent with loss of isotonic fluid such as in hemorrhage, diarrhea, and vomiting.

C: Increase, decrease, increase [Incorrect] This pattern is more consistent with gain of hypotonic fluid such as with water intoxication.

D: Increase, increase, decrease [Correct] This pattern is consistent with hypertonic saline or addition of mannitol.

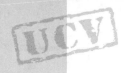

E: Increase, no change, no change [Incorrect] This pattern is more consistent with gain of isotonic fluid.

8.　A

A: Increased alkaline phosphatase levels [Correct] Alkaline phosphotase is indicative of activity of osteoblasts. Osteoblasts are overworking in Paget's disease, and therefore alkaline phosphatase levels will be increased.

B: Decreased calcium levels [Incorrect] This patient has Paget's disease of bone. Calcium levels in this disease are normal. Paget's disease is characterized by abnormal activity of osteoclasts and osteoblasts and usually involves spine, skull, femur, and tibia. Heart failure may occur in early vascular phase of this disease due to many atrioventricular shunts developing in the highly vascular lesions. Hearing loss may come about as a result of narrowing of the auditory foramen.

C: Decreased phosphorus levels [Incorrect] In Paget's disease, phosphorus levels are normal.

D: Decreased alkaline phosphatase levels [Incorrect] Alkaline phosphotase is indicative of activity of osteoblasts. Osteoblasts are overworking in Paget's disease, and therefore alkaline phosphatase levels will be increased, not decreased. Alkaline phosphatase levels may be decreased in osteoporosis.

E: Normal alkaline phosphatase levels [Incorrect] Alkaline phosphatase is indicative of activity of osteoblasts. Osteoblasts are overworking in Paget's disease, and therefore alkaline phosphatase levels will be increased.

9.　C

A: Asthma [Incorrect] While not the most common cause it is common to see pulmonary hypertension secondary to asthma, which is defined as secondary pulmonary hypertension and treatable.

B: Chronic increased oxygen saturation [Incorrect] Increased oxygen saturation dilates pulmonary arteries, leading to decreased resistance to the right heart and less instance of cor pulmonale.

C: Left-sided heart failure [Correct] The most common cause of chronic cor pulmonale is left sided failure with etiologies such as myocardial infarction, longstanding hypertension and alcohol abuse.

D: Myocardial infarction [Incorrect] Heart attacks, as mentioned above, can indirectly lead to right heart pressure overload and hypertrophy that is cor pulmonale.

E: Pulmonary embolism [Incorrect] PE can cause acute cor pulmonale, which refers to right ventricular dilation secondary to increased resistance from the embolus.

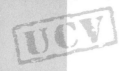
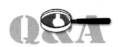

10. C

A: Aortic stenosis results in eccentric hypertrophy of the left ventricle. [Incorrect] Aortic stenosis results in concentric hypertrophy.

B: Mitral regurgitation is associated with a murmur that radiates to the neck. [Incorrect] This is true of aortic stenosis.

C: Mitral regurgitation usually results in a systolic apical murmur that may radiate to the axilla. [Correct] Mitral regurgitation usually results in a systolic murmur best heard at the apex which may radiate to the axilla.

D: Mitral stenosis results in a systolic murmur. [Incorrect] Mitral stenosis results in a diastolic murmur.

E: Pulmonic stenosis results in pulmonary edema. [Incorrect] It is unlikely that pulmonic stenosis will result in pulmonary edema.

11. A

A: Osteopetrosis [Correct] Also known as Albers-Schönberg disease, osteopetrosis occurs due to osteoclast insufficiency. Patients develop multiple fractures due to thickened but structurally weak bone. In addition, anemia may occur secondary to reduced marrow space. Cranial nerve deficits may also arise if nerve impingement occurs in narrowed cranial foramina.

B: Temporal arteritis [Incorrect] This vasculitis is rare in patients younger than 55–60 years of age and typically presents with headache and jaw claudication. Blindness can occur if the disease is not treated.

C: Alport's syndrome [Incorrect] Associated with lens dislocation, sensorineural deafness, platelet defects, and glomerulonephritis, this inherited condition is caused by a defect in collagen. The renal sequelae can be treated by transplantation. Bone is not affected.

D: Diabetes mellitus [Incorrect] Often insidious in its effects, diabetes can cause retinopathy and lens opacification, therefore potentially explaining the patient's vision changes. However, it is not associated with multiple fractures.

E: Iron deficiency anemia [Incorrect] Anemia can explain the fatigue experienced by the patient, but it does not cause the skeletal findings in this case.

12. D

A: Reduced overshoot of the action potential [Incorrect] The overshoot of the action potential is controlled by sodium channels.

B: Reduced duration of the plateau of the action potenial [Incorrect] In fact, the opposite would occur since it would take longer for potassium to cross because of the decreased conductance.

C: Prolonged phase 1 repolarization [Incorrect] Initially, repolarization is controlled by the inactivation of the sodium channels.

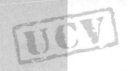

D: Prolonged plateau due to prolongation of phase 2 [Correct] Because the potassium could not have as much conductance due to the defect in the channel, phase 2 of the action potential would be altered.

E: Less negative resting potential [Incorrect] There would be more negative resting potential.

13. A

A: Alpha 1 agonist [Correct] This would increase the sphincter pressure and decrease symptoms of urinary incontinence.

B: Alpha 2 antagonist [Incorrect] This would not have significant impact on the bladder.

C: Beta 2 antagonist [Incorrect] This could contract the bladder and lead to further urinary incontinence.

D: Beta 1 agonist [Incorrect] This could not have significant effect on the bladder. This receptor is found mostly on the heart.

E: Muscarinic agonist [Incorrect] This could contract the bladder increasing symptoms of urinary incontinence.

14. C

A: Acetazolamide [Incorrect] Acetazolamide is a carbonic anhydrase inhibitor. This class of drugs is generally not used to treat hypertension as the diuresis is self limiting within 2–3 days. Mechanism of self-limiting diuresis. By inhibiting carbonic anhydrase in proximal convoluted tubule, acetazolamide causes increased urinary excretion of bicarbonate. As the body bicarbonate level is decreased, excretion slows even with continued diuretic use, and the diuresis becomes self limiting.

B: Amiloride [Incorrect] This is a potassium sparing diuretic. It works in the late distal tubule and the cortical collecting duct by inhibiting Na reabsorption, and K and H secretion. It would be useful for treatment of hypertension. It does not have any effect on reabsorption of calcium. Furosemide is a better answer as it would also help reabsorb calcium to not make the patient's osteoporosis worse.

C: Clorothiazide [Correct] This is a thiazide diuretic that inhibits Na/Cl cotransported in the early distal convoluted tubule. It is useful for treatment of hypertension, especially in a patient with osteoporosis and it increase calcium reabsorption from urine by an unknown mechanism.

D: Furosemide [Incorrect] Furosemide is a loop diuretic that works on medullary ascending loop of Henle by inhibiting Na/K/2Cl cotransport which accounts for 20–25% of reabsorption of Na. Downstream sites cannot compensate for the sodium excretion, which makes these drugs very efficacious and useful for treatment of hypertension. But note that this patient is also suffering from osteoporosis

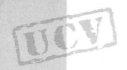 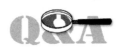

Loop diuretics cause decreased reabsorption of calcium from urine, and may worsen her condition even more. In fact, loop diuretics are often employed for treatment of hypercalcemia (as induced by malignancy for example.)

E: Mannitol [Incorrect] This is an osmotic diuretic. Most of the filtered solutes will be excreted in larger amounts unless they are actively reabsorbed. Osmotic diuretics are not indicated for treatment of hypertension, but may be used to decrease cerebral edema and intraocular pressure.

15. E

A: Decreased calcium, increased phosphate, normal alkaline phosphatase [Incorrect] The above patient has osteoporosis. A patient with decreased calcium, increased phosphate, and normal alkaline phosphatase would most likely present with renal insufficiency.

B: Normal calcium, normal phosphate, increased alkaline phosphatase [Incorrect] A patient with normal calcium, normal phosphate, and increased alkaline phosphatase would not suggest osteoporosis.

C: Increased calcium, decreased phosphate, increased alkaline phosphatase [Incorrect] A patient with increased calcium, decreased phosphate, and increased alkaline phosphatase would not have osteoporosis. This patient could be a candidate for hyperparathyroidism.

D: Increased calcium, increased phosphate, normal alkaline phosphatase [Incorrect] These labs would not suggest osteoporosis. It could, however, suggest Vitamin D intoxication.

E: Normal calcium normal phosphate, normal alkaline phosphatase [Correct] The patient most likely has osteoporosis; therefore, her calcium, phosphate, and alkaline phosphatase would most likely be normal.

16. C

A: A continuous murmur. [Incorrect] Sudden death and an autosomal dominance point strongly to hypertrophic cardiomyopathy (HCM). HCM classically has a systolic crescendo-decrescendo ejection murmur that begins well after S_1. It is often accompanied by the murmur of mitral regurgitation which is a high pitched blowing sounding holosystolic murmur. The description for this answer choice is the murmur of a patent ductus arteriosus.

B: A crescendo-decrescendo systolic ejection murmur beginning immediately after S_1. [Incorrect] A murmur of aortic stenosis is described.

C: A crescendo-decrescendo systolic ejection murmur beginning well after S_1. [Correct] The classic murmur for HCM is described.

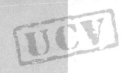

D: High pitched diastolic murmur beginning immediately after S_2 [Incorrect] A murmur of aortic or pulmonary incompetence is described.

E: High pitched systolic murmur beginning well after S_2, often accompanied with an initial snap. [Incorrect] A murmur of mitral stenosis is described.

17. C

A: Inability for the activated vitamin D to bind to the cytosolic receptor in the intestine. [Incorrect] Renal functioning does not change the ability of vitamin D to bind to its cytosolic receptor.

B: Inability to create 7-dehydrocholesterol. [Incorrect] This is a steroid precursor that is not affected by renal function.

C: Inability to make 25-hydroxy 1 hydroxylase. [Correct] This enzyme is decreased in the kidney in chronic renal failure. It is necessary for making 1,25 (OH)2 D3, is the most potent vitamin D metabolite.

D: Inability to make more calcium binding protein once activated vitamin D has changed transcription. [Incorrect] Renal functioning does not change the ability for the receptor-vitamin D complex to cause the calcium binding protein to be made.

E: Inability to make cholecalciferol. [Incorrect] The skin makes vitamin D3 from 7-dehydrocholesterol.

18. C

A: S_1 [Incorrect] While an S_1 may be auscultated in this patient, this is a normal physical exam finding. S_1 occurs when the tricuspid and mitral valve close.

B: S_2 [Incorrect] An S_2 may also be auscultated on this patient; this too is a normal finding. S_2 occurs with pulmonary and aortic valve closure.

C: S_3 [Correct] An S_3 may be auscultated in a patient with dilated congestive heart failure. S_3 occurs at the end of the rapid ventricular filling phase of the cardiac cycle.

D: S_4 [Incorrect] An S_4 would be an abnormal physical exam finding in this patient and is not expected. A S_4 is associated with a hypertrophic ventricle, which would have been noted on the patient's ECHO.

E: Jugular venous distention [Incorrect] JVD is a common finding in patients with right heart failure. There is no evidence of that in this patient.

19. E

A: Sheets of neoplastic cells with keratin pearls [Incorrect] Squamous cell carcinomas metastasize less than 5% of the time, and local excision is curative. Actinic keratoses are precursors to this malignancy

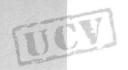

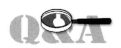

Sun-exposed areas, such as hands, lower lip, and nose, are most often affected.

B: Central connective tissue core under squamous epithelium [Incorrect] Acrochordon, also known as skin tag, is a benign proliferation of normal tissue. This lesion often appears in areas of friction, such as the neck and axillae.

C: Vacuolated cells in the epidermis granular layer [Incorrect] These cells are koilocytes in verucae. Commonly called "warts," papillomavirus causes local proliferation. Human papillomavirus types 16 and 18 are associated with increased risk of cervical cancer.

D: Intertwining bundles of collagen and fibroblasts [Incorrect] This represents the benign finding of dermatofibroma. The cutaneous appearance is that of a firm nodule, possibly demonstrating pigmented acanthosis.

E: Palisading clusters of darkly staining cells [Correct] Basal cell carcinomas are the most common skin cancers. They almost never metastasize. Chronic sun exposure and history of acute sunburn contribute to basal cell carcinoma development.

20. C

A: Continuous machine-like murmur [Incorrect] A continuous machine-like murmur is associated with a patent ductus arteriosis.

B: Crescendo-decrescendo systolic ejection murmur [Incorrect] A crescendo-decrescendo systolic ejection murmur is associated with aortic stenosis.

C: Holosystolic murmur [Correct] A holosystolic murmur is associated with a ventricular septal defect.

D: Late diastolic murmur [Incorrect] A late diastolic murmur is most often found in patients with mitral stenosis.

E: Systolic murmur with a midsystolic click [Incorrect] A systolic murmur with a midsystolic click is most often auscultated on patients with mitral valve prolapse.